INTENTIONAL EATING

AN EASY, MINDFUL APPROACH TO DIETARY WELLNESS FOR INCREASED VITALITY, WEIGHT CONTROL, CHRONIC DISEASE MANAGEMENT AND STRESS REDUCTION

Cyndy Hess deBruler, RPh, CHT

BALBOA.PRESS
A DIVISION OF HAY HOUSE

Balboa Press books may be ordered through booksellers or by contacting:

Balboa Press
A Division of Hay House
1663 Liberty Drive
Bloomington, IN 47403
www.balboapress.com
844-682-1282

Print information available on the last page.

ISBN: 978-1-5043-8843-6 (sc)
ISBN: 978-1-5043-8845-0 (hc)
ISBN: 978-1-5043-8844-3 (e)

Library of Congress Control Number: 2017915222

Balboa Press rev. date: 02/07/2018

Dedicated to my grandson Gage Jun,
My source of joy and inspiration

"Change the way you look at things, and the things you look at change."

— Wayne Dyer, *The Power of Intention*

CONTENTS

INTRODUCTION

Are you living the vital, healthy and fulfilling life you want? Do you eat well and love the foods you eat? Do you sleep well, waking up each day refreshed and energetic, ready for whatever comes your way?

Are you are dealing with weight issues, chronic pain or serious illness? Perhaps you are plagued with stress and fatigue. Maybe you just don't feel good or have the energy you might like. Whatever your wellness level, this book can help.

The path to wellness and a new more vital, healthy life may be easier than you think. My intent is to offer a different way of looking at food and how we eat; a mindful approach that will change your life.

How would your life be different if you had a clear and simple path to a healthier life? Take a moment and imagine what it might be like if you could change. *Why* might you want it to be that way?

The question "*Why?*" is the most important thing to ask yourself right now. Take a minute to think of the reasons *why* you might choose to change your health. Visualize your quality of life *if* you could. *Why* might you want to change your relationship with food? Make a list of these "*whys*" before you start the program for they will determine your willingness to change and give you the support you need when old ways try to creep back in. Keep your list of *"whys"* (perhaps in the "Notes" section in this book) and read and add to them often.

This will be the source of motivation you will need to make these concepts work for you. Maybe you want to feel better about yourself and do things that you cannot now do. Maybe you would change for your kids or grandkids. Think of what matters most to you to find your *"whys"*. (If you cannot identify any *"whys"* right away, keep reading and keep your health in mind.)

Mindful eating is a practice used daily by many Buddhist mindfulness teachers, including Thich Nhat Hanh. This wise and famous Buddhist monk tells a lovely story about being a child and having his mother bring home a single cookie for him in the afternoon. He would take it outside and make that cookie last for hours, eating one bit at a time, relishing the goodness and treasuring the flavor of every bite.

This is a perfect example of mindful or *"intentional eating"*. In Hanh's book Peace Is Every Step, he talks of making every meal a meditation of enjoyment, a ceremony of delight. With the joy in this way of eating comes the added benefit of good health and wellness, especially once you break your food addictions and learn the basics of a good balanced diet that gives your body what you need without all of the bad stuff -- like the sugar, salt and unhealthy fats, or excess quantities.

"You are what you eat," is a quote we hear a lot. It cannot be taken literally to mean, "If you eat a shrimp, you are a shrimp," but looking to the quote's real roots reveals some great wisdom. This shortened version of the quote probably came from the French gastronome, Jean Anthelme Brillat-Savarin in his statement, "Tell me what you eat and I shall tell you what you are." This quote actually makes more sense. So what, exactly, are you eating? Fruits and vegetables? Fast food? Gourmet? Exotic? Ethnic? Do you eat real foods prepared naturally? Whether you are a gourmet chef or don't know how to cook, this book can show you ways to eat and feel better.

The type of food you choose to consume is a direct reflection of the kind of person you are, as well as a reflection of your life experiences and choices. These foods are also a reflection of your state of health, the vitality you have, and how good you feel. What you choose to put into your mouth today will determine who, and how healthy you are tomorrow. Do you want to wake up every day well rested, feeling great, with the energy you need to really enjoy your life? It is all in *what* you eat and *how* you eat it.

Did you know french fries and iceberg lettuce are the two most widely consumed vegetables in America? Is it any wonder that over two-thirds of Americans are overweight, with the average American carrying 23 pounds more than their target weight? Of these, more than 30% are clinically obese.

This extra weight we carry has now been linked to increases in most chronic diseases including diabetes, heart disease, cancer, and Alzheimers. Diabetes doubles the risk of getting Alzheimers Disease! According to the United States Healthful Food Council, "Many experts believe that improved nutrition and lifestyle can reduce illnesses and deaths from cancer by as much as 40%, death from cardiovascular disease by up to 30%, and cases of diabetes by at least 50%. Unfortunately, America is moving in the wrong direction. Since 1990, diabetes has increased 61%, obesity 75%.

Heart disease is now the number one killer of adults and **second leading cause of death for children under 15!"**

Over the past 25 years, the number of overweight adults has doubled. The number of overweight children has more than tripled. Life expectancies are dramatically decreasing in one of the most "advanced" countries in the world.

There are many healthy lifestyle approaches being promoted now. These include eating organic whole foods, eating a Paleo diet, eating vegetarian or vegan, eating low-glycemic, Mediterranean, "clean eating", etc. These movements are getting away from the older idea of calorie counting "diets". The shift away from calorie counting reflects our understanding that dieting with limited portions and calorie counting has been shown to fail over 95% of the time.

Traditional diets just don't work for most people as they are based on what *you can't have* and that is a proven recipe for rebound binge and post-diet overeating. *Food should be a pleasurable experience, not one of denial.* Many of the new approaches listed above are vast improvements from the calorie counting diets, but they often miss *changing your relationship to food* through how you eat. This critical missing element is what I call *"intentional eating"*.

As the lifestyle of people across the planet has become more and more hectic, with longer work-weeks and increased stress, the average American family eats more fast food meals. They are ubiquitous, convenient and involve less time and planning. A surprising 40% of the American family's food budget is spent on eating out, so the price adds up quickly. Add a couple of dinners at a real restaurant and voila — not so cheap. Fast foods are extensively marketed to the public, especially our children, to the point *addictions* to the taste of sugar, salt and fat are the driving force behind most peoples' eating decisions.

The national average for fast food meals is four to six times a week per person. It may be hard to believe but 30% percent of our children eat at least one fast food meal daily. When people do eat at home, it is often processed foods and microwaved dinners. Most pre-packaged meals are severely lacking in nutritional value but loaded in sugar, bad fats and artificial flavorings. What they lack in nutrition, they make up for in ease of preparation. We throw them in the microwave (and kill off any remaining live nutrients and all enzymes, crucially needed by our bodies for good health.)

On top of these realities, an increasing number of families are economically challenged by the ever-rising prices of food, especially vegetables, fruits, and meats. It becomes difficult to make the tough decision to cook meals from scratch using fresh vegetables and good quality proteins. Working long hours, possibly two or more jobs, and just trying to raise a family with all the hustle and bustle of the American lifestyle make meal planning, preparation and cleanup just too much. Furthermore, very few people were taught about nutrition or how important it is to the health of their families. We are tired, stressed out, grossly overweight, but sadly under-nourished. The consequences are becoming more and more evident and dire.

So how do we take back our lives and regain our health? Perhaps we start by gaining some basic knowledge about the nutrition we need and the food choices available to us. Then, by becoming aware of the addictive nature of most of our eating choices, we consciously choose to break the addictions controlling us. (Usually this requires a cleanse, reboot or fasting to reset our body's metabolism and take away the addictive signals from our brains.) Finally, we make a conscious decision to become more aware of eating and truly listening to our body's needs. Our new life style requires thinking and planning. It requires *attention* to what we buy and eat daily, then *intention* or mindfulness with every bite. The pleasures and rewards are well worth the effort.

If we do not change the way we eat, the consequences will be very serious, both personally and as a society. My goal is to provide a concise overview of what you need to know to get started on your journey with food. Once we learn what foods are healthy, how often we should eat, and in which amounts and combinations, then we can begin to find a way to make the right choices daily, until they are an integral part of who we are.

While *"intentional eating"* is the guiding principle that will bring you to the right foods for you, **until you are able to break the addictions, you cannot clearly make the right food choices.** You may wish to come back and reread Chapter 3 once you have completed the Reboot Program. *Then* you will be able to begin to listen to your body and eat with intention.

When we bring mindfulness or *intention* into the process of eating, we pause and observe the INTENT we have with every mouthful we chose, the foods we eat will change. Healthy eating will become a habit and the joy of eating will return as our taste buds come alive again, and we eat with intention and focus on each bite. Mealtime will offer genuine joy, not the addictive fix that comes from the taste of sugar or fat. It will not happen overnight, but it is possible and really quite easy.

There is a knowing in each of our bodies of what is good for us and what is not.

Your first active step is to break the cycle of food addictions and reset your metabolism to maintain healthy blood sugar levels throughout the day. Then your body can guide you to the wholesome nourishment in a diet comprised of mostly fresh fruits and vegetables, with adequate quality protein and healthy oils of your choosing. You are on the way to improved health and wellness.

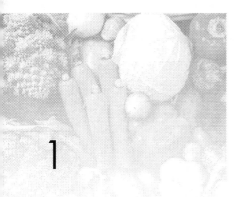

1

Breaking the Cycle of Addiction

Our culture is prone to addiction. We are addicted to drugs, alcohol, smoking, food, shopping, sex, Sunday football…you name it. Almost everyone has some sort of addiction. We seem to depend upon and even subconsciously *enjoy* these addictions as they provide a much needed source of identity, comfort and sense of self.

Within the addicted psyche, there is a sense of "lack". That sense of lack drives consumption as we seek to fill the void with something to soothe us. Sometimes it is alcohol or drugs. Often it is food. Some foods are more likely to be addictive. Sugar, fat, and salt are the worst offenders. The huge food and drug corporations have basically used these poisons to control our food purchasing and fatten their bottom line. The most profitable aisle of the grocery store happens to be the cereal section where tons of cheap, low-quality grains are loaded with sugars, coloring and flavorings to appeal to the youngest of shoppers and feed a growing sugar addiction in the most vulnerable, our children. The Big Food Industry is causing a health crisis across the planet.

Take a minute and imagine, if you will, a big pile of cauliflower or a mountain of apple slices. Do you know anyone that would binge on the cauliflower or apple slices? When you change the image to a pile of cookies or a mountain of potato chips, the response changes. It becomes easy to imagine someone who cannot help eating the last chip or munching all the cookies. Let's look at what the difference is between these two scenarios.

Many doctors and nutritional specialists believe it is caused by a certain irresistible combination of sugar, fats, and salt. Some experts believe that 'food science' has perfected this toxic combining to make saying no to these addictive foods extremely difficult, if not impossible. Volatile chemical compounds assault our taste buds with artificial flavorings to make even "low sugar" foods taste sweet and the chips with low sodium levels taste salty. Everything has more flavor, actually dulling our taste buds to the point that healthy foods may taste bland and undesirable. Fresh vegetables and fruits are certainly not something you want to grab when you need a pick-me-up or a mood changer.

<u>Sugar Blues</u>, a book written in 1975 by William Duffy, documents how we became addicted to sugar. The process is the same for salt and fats. We are talking physical addiction here folks...just like the addiction caused by heroin! What is just becoming apparent now is the extent of the biological and very real food addiction that people who are overweight or eat unhealthy foods experience. Addiction is a disease and choice or

restraint is not an option. It must be treated and the addiction healed.

"Sugar is the biggest public health crisis in the history of the world," says Dr. Robert Lustig, an endocrinologist at the University of California, San Francisco. His 2009 speech "Sugar: The Bitter Truth" has received more than 2.5 million hits on YouTube. In a paper published in 2015 in the journal *Nature*, Lustig and his colleagues provoked debate when they stated that sugar is so harmful, it should be regulated like alcohol and tobacco. "Every substance of abuse — cocaine, heroin, you name it — has required personal or social intervention," says Lustig. "For sugar we have nothing, and my prediction is that we will need both."

Let's look at sugar addiction briefly, as it is the primary culprit on which the others rely.

Sugar in all its forms is the root cause of our obesity epidemic and most of the chronic disease sucking the life out of American citizens and the economy (and increasingly the world). You name it; it's caused by sugar. Heart disease, cancer, dementia, type 2 diabetes, anxiety, depression. Even acne, infertility, impotence, and Alzheimers have all been linked to obsessive sugar intake.

You cannot win by reading labels, as there are dozens of names for hidden sugars. Processed foods rarely have just one sugar, but many, and most are disguised under strange unfamiliar names we would never think of for sugar. Names we don't recognize like erythritol, barley malt, dextrose, maltose, sucrose, brown rice syrup, fruit juice concentrate and on and on. The average American consumes over 150 pounds of sugars a year!

That's roughly 22 teaspoons every day for every person in

America. In addition, our kids consume about 34 teaspoons (that's more than two 20-ounce sodas a day) making nearly one in four teenagers pre-diabetic or diabetic.

Sadly, (because we all love a great loaf of bread) **flour is nothing more than another form of sugar because it is metabolized quickly into sugar in the body.** Grains are a fairly new addition to the human diet and not a good one. Eating flour in breads and pastas compounds the sugars we get from processed foods and baked goods. Americans consume about 146 pounds of flour a year. An important but unknown fact is that **flour raises blood sugar *even more* than table sugar** because of how it is digested in the body. This is true for almost all flours, even whole-wheat and whole-grain flours. Estimates for sugar consumption are between 150-170 pounds per year per American. If we stop to think about it – that's 296 pounds per year for both using the lower estimate. That is just under one pound of sugar and flour ***consumed daily*** for every man, woman and child in America!

Here's a shocking fact: sugar is eight times as physically addictive as cocaine! In tests, rats will choose sugar water over food, sex and any other substance until it kills them.

Sugar in all its forms **(including flour)** is the reason nearly 70 percent of Americans and 40 percent of kids are overweight. In one study, Harvard scientists found that a high sugar milkshake (compared to a low sugar one) not only spiked blood sugar and insulin and led to more sugar cravings, but caused huge changes in the brain. The sugar lit up the addiction center called the *nucleus accumbens* in the brain. These biological changes are easy to see and measure with brain scans and blood tests. They are real!

Do you have pre-diabetes or type 2 diabetes? Ninety percent of these disorders go undiagnosed. Do you have belly fat? Are you overweight? Crave sugar and carbs? Have trouble losing weight? Have you been measured with high triglycerides, low HDL or been told your blood sugar is a "little high"? In some countries, diabetes is simply called 'Sugar'.

Do you eat when you are not hungry or experience a food-induced sleepiness after eating? Do you feel bad about your eating habits or avoid certain activities because of your eating? Do you get withdrawal symptoms like dizziness, fatigue or headaches if you cut down or stop sugar or carbs? Perhaps you need more and more of the same bad foods just to feel good? These are all symptoms of health sabotaging sugar (and carb) addiction.

Food addiction is not a simple emotional eating disorder as the food industry would like you to believe! Stop feeling guilty! It is a biological disorder and a true addiction. Out of balance hormones and neurotransmitters in our bodies fuel sugar and carb cravings, leading to uncontrolled overeating and consumption of substances that should not be considered food.

The big three big food addictions are sugar, fat, and salt. While sugar may be the worst, unhealthy fats and too much salt and flavorings are right behind in creating an unhealthy planet. They can be found in abundance in most processed foods and almost all fast foods. How many people do you know who sit at home at night and will have a cookie or several, followed by something salty, then something containing fat like ice cream?

It becomes a vicious cycle and the practice of eating mindlessly while watching TV makes it worse. Dr. Dean Ornish, a pioneer in nutrition and health, makes the case that the first bite of ice cream is always the best. So why don't we stop there? Realistically, most of us cannot -- no more than the heroin addict can say no to the next fix.

The Food Industry and the American government encourage more "personal responsibility." Their answer to the crisis in obesity and health related illness is individuals exercising self-control, making better choices, avoiding over-eating and just reducing your intake of sugar-sweetened drinks. They lead us to believe there is no good food or bad food. It is only a matter of balance and calories. Just eat less and exercise more. This sounds good in theory, but new scientific studies prove that industrial processed, fat, sugar and salt-laden food is addictive. Apples are not addictive, nor is broccoli or kale, but soda, chips, and cookies can absolutely become addictive drugs. Self-control and increased exercise are not the solutions.

It is as hard for the biologically-addicted person to drive by their favorite fast food place, or take a small bowl of ice cream and not follow it with something else or more of the same, as it is for a cocaine addict or a drunk to "just say no." Addiction is a *disease* that needs to be healed like any other if you are to move beyond it. Food addiction is no different. People don't want to be fat. They usually know what they are doing is destructive but they cannot stop. It is interesting that many people go through a "healing crisis" with physical side effects when they stop eating these foods, just as the caffeine junkie gets headaches or the alcoholic gets the shakes.

New studies show that sugar stimulates the brain's reward

centers through the neurotransmitter dopamine exactly like other addictive drugs. Brain scans show that high-sugar, high-fat foods and even artificial sweeteners work just like heroin, opium, or morphine in the brain. Obese people and drug addicts both have lower numbers of dopamine receptors, making it more likely to crave things that boost dopamine in the brain.

Furthermore, foods high in fat and sweets stimulate the release of the body's own opioids or "feel good" chemicals in the brain. This has been further documented by studies showing that the brain's receptors for heroin and morphine are the same receptors involved in preference for sweet, high fat foods in both normal and over-weight eaters.

Just like with other addictions, people and rats develop a tolerance to sugar, needing more and more to satisfy themselves. Moreover, we all know obese individuals continue to eat large amounts of unhealthy foods despite severe personal health and social consequences. Just like other addicts, humans on soda pop addictions will experience "withdrawal" symptoms when cut off. They need the food or sugary drink to just feel normal long after the initial period of enjoyment has passed and many people drink pop or diet soda in massive quantities.

A Harvard Study published in the Journal of the American Medical Association showed that overweight adolescents consumed an extra 500 calories on average daily when allowed to eat junk food as compared to days when junk food was not allowed. They ate more food because the *food itself triggered the cravings and addictive reaction.* Sugar, fat, and salt stimulated their brain's reward centers. They wanted more and could not stop.

So what does the Big Food Industry have to say about these new studies? They keep coming back to the three refrains used over and over. They state: 1) It is all about personal choice. Government regulation on how you market or what you can offer to eat violates civil liberties and should not be tolerated, 2) There are no good foods or bad foods. It is solely about amount, so no specific foods can be blamed for the obesity epidemic, 3) We need to focus on education about exercise not diet, because it shouldn't matter what you eat if you burn off those calories. This is merely propaganda from an industry that relies on the profits from a high number of addicted people eating mass-marketed processed food, not one interested in nourishing the nation or the world. And of course, the huge drug industry and medical institutions also benefit more from a sick population. We are only seeing the tip of the iceberg with the health care industry crisis with lots of money to be made by the very industry charged with improving our health.

Unfortunately, industrial food giant corporations control school lunchrooms and encourage our young folk to consume sports drinks now (loaded with sugars) instead of pop. Indeed, they control our entire food chain from industrialized farming to the grocery store and restaurant. According to one estimate, fifty percent of meals are eaten outside the home. Many home cooked meals are simple microwavable industrial food. There is no clear labeling and all efforts to get effective labeling are energetically combated with big money. Few people know that an order of cheese fries is 2,900 calories or an afternoon latte can be over 500 calories.

Huge changes are needed at the political level to increase healthy food availability and make it affordable for the average American. The "eat local" and farmer's market movements are part of the answer, but it is a story of David vs. Goliath. In the meantime, we do need to take personal responsibility, not to limit calories, but to break the addictions in ourselves and our children. I hope you are convinced. If not, do the research for yourself. There is a serious problem here. We must break free of nutritionally empty foods filling our grocery stores that harm our bodies and destroy our health.

So how do we do that?

My recommended method for how to break food addictions is covered in detail in Chapter 2. It is a very simple Reboot Program that anyone can do in 10 days. Yes, it requires commitment, but you can eat five meals a day without limiting portions (within reason), and you will feel satisfied. It will allow you to begin losing significant weight, lower and normalize your blood sugar levels, lower your blood pressure, lower your bad cholesterol and become a new healthier you. **Are you ready?**

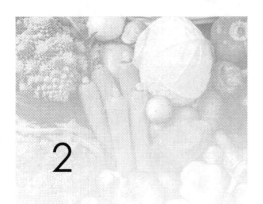

2
Rebooting Your Metabolism

▬▬ ▬▬ ▬▬ ▬▬ ▬▬ ▬▬

"The most important decision we make is whether we believe we live in a friendly or hostile universe."

— Albert Einstein

Food is not your enemy. Finding the right foods and learning to enjoy and find delight in eating healthy foods is the task at hand.

As a pharmacist and nutritional counselor, I have studied nutrition and various diets for more than 20 years. I've taught many weight loss classes and for years saw mixed results. Every body is different and what works for one often fails for another. Some people can lose weight and feel better by eating animal proteins and vegetables and limiting carbs. Some people do much better without any meat protein, choosing vegetables and healthy whole grains, seeds and nuts. Without eliminating the addictions first, either way is doomed to eventual failure. Diets restricting calories do not work. Anytime we restrict ourselves in eating volume or calories, there usually is a rebound price to pay. Statistics show that over 90% regain more than weight they have lost.

So what does work? First, we need to do a Reboot to **reset your metabolism and break the addictions**. You may have heard about some programs for rebooting your metabolism as many doctors and wellness advocates are now endorsing it. Sometimes there are problems with the way it is presented: 1) it is too difficult, 2) it requires you buying expensive supplements only they sell, 3) there are no specific meal plan guidelines that most of us can easily integrate into our busy lifestyle.

The Reboot can be accomplished by following the guidelines in this book's Appendix, or if you prefer, by juicing with vegetables and some fruits for a period of time. Juicing offers the benefits of a reboot for your metabolism and breaks addiction. But for many people, juicing alone has little appeal or feels impossible. So what is this new way to overcome the addictions without fasting or juicing or calorie counting?

First, the good news! You can eat as much as you need and as often as you like with the Reboot Program in this book! Most people find the Reboot phase of eating quite easy and satisfying once they get through the occasionally difficult first couple of days.

We change our bodies, our metabolism, and our relationship to food by going "cold turkey" to the addictive substances in our foods for the 10-day period. Anyone who truly wants a healthier body and better life can do without these foods for 10 days if they can eat freely and regularly and feel satisfied. I will show you how and assure you that at the end of the 10 days, you will feel radically changed. You will not want sugary foods and even cheese may seem just too thick and fatty for your new palate. Gradually, you may add some of the foods back into your diet, but in moderation or as occasional treats, not regular fare. Basically you will be eating whole foods, mostly plant based with an adequate amount of the protein right for you.

Please see the Reboot Program Guide in the Appendix for specifics on what you should and should not eat as well as ideas on what to snack on and how to make a satisfying meal from allowable foods. In the Reboot, you are going to eat five times a day or at least every three hours. If you are used to three meals a day, like most of us, you are going to add snacks in between these meals. If you are someone who often skips meals, you have to make the time and eat regularly. With no quantity limits and eating frequently, you will move forward without great distress if you make the commitment. It helps greatly to have a partner or your family's participation. Support and accountability are crucial.

There are "forbidden foods" for the ten days including all forms of added sugars, artificial sweeteners, alcohol, limited caffeine, and all processed foods. You are going to eat simply from whole natural foods that nourish and begin the healing process. When I first did the 10-day Reboot, I had blood tests from my doctor before and after. My blood sugar level dropped 20 points, my cholesterol dropped 40 points, and my blood pressure normalized about ten points below what it had been. In 10 days!

All my parameters were within "normal limits" before the Reboot. For me, it was fun to see the radical change 10 days could make in my blood chemistry! (If you have any serious chronic illnesses, it is highly recommended you only do the Reboot Phase under the supervision of your MD or naturopathic physician.)

The first three days can be a challenge. Most people will have to be quite disciplined during the first few days to keep it together. We find out we are so accustomed to indulging ourselves to feed our addictions. It may be best not to have the most tempting non-allowed foods in the house. Clean out your cupboards and refrig before you start. The cravings may be challenging. Minor health discomforts, such as like slight headaches and just not feeling good, are not uncommon. These are often described as "detox" reactions as our bodies begin to cleanse. The good news: it is all downhill from here and you will soon feel good and find it easy and satisfying.

Many people are surprised how easy it is not to drink alcohol perhaps fearing it would be the hardest part. Wrong, after the first few days, you won't even miss it. Maybe you don't believe you can make it through the afternoon at work without that diet Coke, but it's worth the effort. I recommend substituting a glass of sparkling water or coconut water with mint or lime for those times when a special beverage is desired like after work or before or after dinner. There are so many psychological ways we use food to get through our stress-filled days, that you will begin to *notice* the habits and rituals that have become part of our lives. Perhaps the ice cream at night will be the toughest part. We reward ourselves with food so leaving these rewards behind or substituting healthy ones may be challenging at first.

This is why I recommend being **absolutely strict** for the first 10 days. Your body will do fine and after day three, it will be easier because you will start to notice differences. You can do it!

If you suffer from serious chronic diseases, it is important to see your doctor before beginning the Reboot Program. This is especially important if you are diabetic or suffer from other blood sugar level disorders. Your need for medication may change during your reboot quite quickly. What will happen as you follow the Reboot Program is your blood sugar will balance and maintain a more stable level throughout the day. There will be fewer spikes in your insulin level and your body will begin to find metabolic stability. This is the factor that allows for the large weight loss many people experience in this phase even though they are eating more often and as much as they want of the allowable foods. Because you are eating at least five times a day, you will naturally eat smaller amounts and be satisfied. The foods you eat are nutrient-rich and wholesome. After a few days of addiction withdrawal, you will feel better than you have in a long time.

You will begin each day with a nutritious breakfast with protein. It may be a protein shake or eggs with veggies. No bagels or cereal, no sugary pastries or protein bars. The guidelines of what to eat are specific and if you follow them closely, it will be easy to make the right food choices. Planning ahead and having the right foods on hand is key. My husband relied on veggie sticks and hummus and always had a bag of washed and cut celery in the fridge. A good supply of raw unsalted nuts is another important staple you will want on hand. Hard-boiled eggs are a good snack and easy to carry to work or play. If possible, I highly recommend adding a green drink to your diet, perhaps as your afternoon snack. It will give you more energy than a soda with caffeine and is very filling so it will help you to eat less at dinner and be fully satisfied. Any kind of juicer will work, but I have found the NutriBullet to be a great little investment if you don't have a Vitamix. It is easy to use and wash allowing your entire juicing process to be about five minutes from refrigerator through cleanup.

If you have chronic stomach problems or experience allergic reactions, you may choose to eliminate foods known to be the primary sources of food allergies for the 10-day cleanse and reboot. Often food allergies will trigger cravings. The basic food plan does not prohibit some of these foods so you may want to try an alternative like the UltraSimple Diet or Virgin Diet if you suspect food allergies.

It is important to get adequate sleep during the 10-day cleanse and reboot as inadequate hours of sleep can increase cravings and decrease your body's ability to heal.

Use supplemental craving control if necessary. There are a multitude of supplements available but be careful not to choose ones with artificial sweeteners or stimulants like guarana or caffeine in them. Some of the supplements that help are glutamine, tyrosine, and 5-HTP (amino acids that help reduce cravings). Chromium or other blood sugar balancers like cinnamon can help and glucomannan fiber can reduce spikes in sugar and insulin. Green coffee bean extract or green tea extract also can be helpful.

There are two supplements I strongly advise people do use during the cleanse. Start each day with a fiber or colon cleanse, preferably in a drink followed by a full glass of water. Have the same colon cleanse mix before bed. Choose one that is psyllium-based without an herbal laxative in it. The second supplement is a good digestive enzyme that you take 20 minutes before eating your main meals (lunch and dinner). We are all lacking in enzymes. They are our body's catalysts for every chemical reaction in us, crucial in absorbing and utilizing nutrition from your food.

Drinking water is also key. Lots of water throughout the day but ***never with a meal***. Drinking water or anything else with meals dilutes your stomach acid and prevents proper digestion. See the guide on how and when to drink your water in the Reboot Program Guide. If we are drinking enough water, our urine should be clear.

Most important, don't give up! You can and will make it through the 10-day Reboot and feel happier, stronger and more vital.

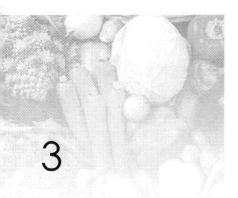

3

Bringing INTENTION to Eating

▬ ▬ ▬ ▬ ▬ ▬

"Drink your tea slowly and reverently, as if it is the axis on which the world earth revolves - slowly, evenly, without rushing toward the future. Live the actual moment. Only this moment is life."

— Thich Nhat Hanh

One could add -- eat your food slowly and reverently as well!

My inspiration for this book was a moment when I was drinking a green drink I had concocted from various vegetables and fruits in my refrigerator. Finding such delight in the flavors as I drank it, I realized it was not only good for me, it was a real treat. I thought that if more people ate totally *in the moment with intention and awareness*, they could more easily eat well and experience better health and quality of life as a result.

Mindfulness seems to have two pillars: intention and attention. If we are aware that we want to live with kindness and love towards ourselves and our bodies, as well as towards others, we carry that knowing as intention. We intend to treat our body as if our health and wellness is ultimately important to us and that guides our eating choices. Then we must attend to the intention with attention. We must pay attention to what foods we eat by planning and making careful choices that honor that intention.

Think about every mouthful of food as an answer to this question: "Is this food really who I am and the health I choose for my body?"

When we eat with such mindfulness, I believe we will learn to make better food choices. Of course, we must have basic knowledge of what foods our body needs and how to make them readily available to us when we are hungry. We need to take the time to plan our meals and buy real food so that our pantry and refrigerator are stocked with good natural, unprocessed foods. Then, with the intent to treat our bodies well for health and vitality, we can pay attention to what we put together for a meal.

If we are eating out, we will choose a restaurant that serves foods that are natural, wholesome and vital, perhaps one where organic foods are available or where the chef takes the time to shop for local meats and vegetables. Even a meal eaten "on the run" can be relaxing and enjoyable moment by moment, if we relish the flavors and tasty goodness. Always take adequate time to eat. When we are finished eating, off we go, but perhaps more mindful of the moment and at a bit slower pace than before the meal that brought us into more mindful awareness.

Perhaps mindfulness is a new concept to you. It is an effort to be more aware and present in every moment of life as we experience it. Instead of thinking about where we have to be in an hour or worrying about who is picking the kids up after school, we take life as it comes, living every minute as fully and presently as possible. Applying this to food and eating, we taste the food fully and have a greater awareness of the act of eating.

We take the time to plan what we eat and we take the time to feel gratitude before eating. We enjoy the company we are with and all of our senses are fully engaged and livened by the experience. Mindfulness allows for seeing more clearly and realizing how the choices we make every moment determine the quality of our lives. Practicing acting with intention and mindfulness offers an opportunity to step away from habitual and reactive patterns.

Practicing mindfulness does not require any previous skills or beliefs. Anyone can do it at any moment. It is always there, waiting for us to slow down and smell the garlic. Perhaps you will also smell the rose in a beautiful vase at the table. The rose is there for a reason, to engage the senses of sight and smell, making the eating experience more enjoyable. It is up to us to choose to look at it or smell it or to be in too much of a hurry to even notice it is there.

Imagine eating a meal at McDonalds. It is often noisy, hectic and we may quickly throw down our meal of burgers, fries and a soft drink without ever really tasting the food. It is a mindless activity, not a mindful one. Our minds are elsewhere, perhaps on the game we are going to or the work yet to be completed that day.

If you want experiential proof, I challenge you to eat very healthy for just two days with fresh seasonal fruit to start the day, then lots of fresh vegetables, salads for lunch, smaller servings of meats, fewer carbs, and little or no processed food. Then go to McDonalds and order the fast food meal. Slowly unwrap the burger and take a bite. Slowly chew it and really focus on what you taste. Maybe it will be a relief and welcome treat (if you are severely addicted to fats and sugars), but more than likely that big bun will be tasteless, white fluff and the rest of the burger will not be anything you really enjoy.

In just a short time without bad foods, your taste buds come back to life. The fast food meal is not what you remembered the meal to taste like before and you just cannot enjoy it when you concentrate on it slowly pay attention to the taste and textures, how it feels in your mouth and your stomach. You have just done a mini cleanse, giving your taste buds a break from sugars, fats and salty processed foods and in just two days, your relationship with food has changed.

If you want vibrant health, loads of energy and freedom from disease and digestive problems or perhaps a slimmer waistline, you can do this same type of cleanse for 10 days or even two weeks. The simple guidelines are in this book. By making an effort to "reboot" your senses and your metabolism, by being very intentional and aware of the foods you eat for just this short time, I truly believe you will make better choices and see a whole new relationship with food develop. If you follow these guidelines, healthy eating is not accomplished because you want to be healthy, but because it tastes better and resonates with what your body wants and needs for life.

Are you eating quickly without thought? Perhaps hurrying between errands? Standing up, reading the paper or watching TV?

How you eat and how much intention and attention you give to the practice of eating, as it matters right now in the moment, is the key to balance and health. Bringing mindfulness and intention to eating is delightful and enriches our lives.

Once you try it, you will be hooked. Not because it is good for you, but because it is delightful and fun. Enjoy your food and enjoy your company and surroundings. Make them matter because the present moment is all that really matters in our life experiences.

The benefits to eating and living with intention and attention include:

- Becoming less hurried and less stressed in every aspect of life
- Becoming more present and enjoying life more
- Becoming more self-aware and feeling more connections with the world and others
- Learning who you truly are
- Learning to distinguish between oneself and one's thoughts
- Learning to let go of worry and guilt, which have no place in the present moment
- Creating greater self-acceptance and compassion towards yourself and others
- Experiencing vitality and health you may have never dreamed possible

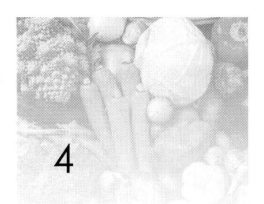

4

What Foods Our Bodies Need

Other than air and lots of water (our bodies are 60-70% water), our most basic nutritional needs are in six basic nutrient groups. These are in two categories known as macronutrients (including proteins, carbohydrates, and fats) and micronutrients (including vitamins, minerals, and phytonutrients.)

It is important to note that not all foods are equal in nutrient content. Only real foods, naturally high in nutritional content and minimally processed, can provide our bodies with what they need to be healthy. Locally grown organic fruits and vegetables, clean complete proteins (whether meat based or of a vegetarian source), and healthy oils are the foods we need to be putting into our bodies for optimal nutrition.

There are a few principles of healthy eating that are common to all of the best food eating styles. Our diets should be mostly plant based. Those plants should be eaten as soon after harvest as possible as nutritional value declines rapidly with real foods. All foods should be minimally processed, only lightly cooked or raw (exceptions are meat and fish).

Avoid gluten. Even if you are not gluten intolerant, it has been shown to cause or increase various health issues. It is possible that the newly developed strains of wheat are harder for our bodies to digest so look for heirloom wheat called Einkorn if you must consume any wheat products. For more information on why and how to avoid gluten, I highly recommend reading the book <u>Grain Brain</u> by Dr. Perlletter.

Because of the extreme impact of high glycemic foods on our insulin levels and overall health, simple carbohydrates like sugars, flours and processed white foods should be eaten only on rare occasions or as treats. Flour has the same or worse impact on our bodies as pure sugar so eating with that in mind is extremely wise, decreasing or **eliminating most if not all flours**. Read labels closely and do not buy foods with added sugars or gluten. (Remember there are many names for hidden sugars and over 40 names for gluten.) The fewer ingredients the better in most instances. Choose grains with the lowest glycemic levels as they are the healthiest. Quinoa and black rice are two good choices. Even if you are vegetarian, focus on more protein and fats in place of carbohydrates including nuts, seeds, coconut, avocados and good oils. Starchy beans should be eaten sparingly.

Good oils are the ones that are high in omega 3 fats. Stay away from the various commonly encountered vegetable oils including canola, sunflower, corn, soy and palm oils. They are all high in omega 6 oils which are not good for us. Instead focus on olive oil, coconut oil, avocado oil, nut oils and even saturated fats like butter from uncontaminated grass fed sources.

If you choose to eat meat or fish, do your research and buy the cleanest, most uncontaminated products available. Grass fed, organic meat and dairy is the best choice. Most people who do eat meat eat too much of it. Sustainable fish is a better choice if available where you live as it is higher in omega oils and easy to digest. Reduce the amount in your diet to benefit your body and the planet. Eat healthy vegetarian meals for at least a couple days of the week. (Eating lower on the food chain has a much lessor impact on the environment than eating animal protein.)

Drink an abundance of water at the right times. (See Appendix for more info on specifics but please remember don't consume water with your meals.) It is also important to NEVER drink cold or icy beverages of any kind with meals as cold beverages make digestion very difficult solidifying oils and decreasing absorption of nutrients.

The quality of the food we put into our bodies may be more important than what we eat. Buy and consume fresh, whole foods as they will nourish your body the best. When we digest our food, our metabolic system carries these nutrients to our cells. These nutrients comprise the structure of the cells of our bodies and define our state of health.

If we eat unhealthy and toxic foods, our cells become unhealthy and toxic. Our cells are the building blocks of our bodies. Toxic food equals toxic bodies and minds. Malnutrition and toxic waste buildup are the causes of disease in our bodies. Adequate nutrition, detoxing and digestion are the key to good health. According to Dr. Joseph Mercola, *"Eighty percent of your immune system is located in your digestive system, making a healthy gut a major focal point if you want to maintain optimal health."* This is why what and how you eat are so crucial, not only to your weight, but to your whole body and mind health.

There is a great deal of new information out now on what is called the microbiome. It is the entire system of life that lives in us and on us including viruses, an abundance of various bacteria and a multitude of other microorganisms including troublesome parasites that infest our bodies when we are out of balance. It has been said that for every single cell in our bodies, there are 10,000 microorganisms that also abide in us and on us. While commonly believed and quoted, this is probably a high estimate and it is more likely we have just slightly more microorganisms than cells. But at 37 trillion estimated human cells, it hardly matters. It still is a huge factor regardless.

The state of our particular microbiome is what really determines our overall health, including how well our digestive and immune systems work. Prebiotics are said by many to be even more important in balancing this complex codependent system than the popular probiotics. Probiotics are taken to reestablish healthy bacteria in our gut. They are especially important after taking any antibiotics where gut bacteria may be harmed. Prebiotics are found in fermented foods, the pulp of citrus and other plant based sources. With adequate prebiotics and good plant based nutrition, we can establish and maintain a happy, healthy microbiome and have optimal health.

Proteins:

Protein from food is broken down by the digestive system into amino acids -- the building blocks of life. They are used for building and repairing cells, muscles, hair, and other tissues and for making hormones. Adequate protein intake is important for a healthy immune system. Primary sources of protein are animal products (like meat, fish, poultry, and dairy) and vegetable sources (like beans, lentils, nuts, and seeds). The amount of protein you need varies depending on your body type and fitness level but is probably *much less* than what you are currently eating, especially if you are a meat eater. We do not need quarter pounders, and in fact, too much protein can be very hard on us creating toxin buildup in the gut.

Carbohydrates:

Carbohydrates are plant-based in origin and are a primary source of energy. Carbohydrates consist of two types: simple and complex. Simple carbohydrates are sugars or foods that break down into sugars in the body immediately and have a high glycemic index (GI) like white flour and white rice, meaning they cause your blood sugar to spike more than foods with a lower glycemic index. After your blood sugar level spikes, it usually falls quickly causing fatigue or other symptoms. Complex carbohydrates are comprised of dietary fiber and starch and include whole grains, nuts, fruits, and have a lower glycemic index because they take more time to break down in the body and be digested.

Certain foods have higher or lower glycemic indexes by nature. Charts can be found online if you want to avoid high glycemic fruits and vegetables for the most optimal control of blood sugar and maximum weight loss. Flours, cereals and other refined carbohydrates have typically the highest GI's and really need to be avoided as much as possible. With carbohydrates, quantity or serving size is also important. When amount is considered, you get glycemic load (GL) which some believe more important than GI.

As with some "bad" fats, some sources of carbohydrates can be pro-inflammatory. The glycemic index and glycemic load are indicators of the oxidative stress that will occur as a result of ingesting certain foods. Simple carbohydrates provide calories and short-term energy, but no nutrition. As you eat more high-GI foods, such as breads, white potatoes, pasta, sugars, chips, crackers and snack foods, your body processes these foods as simple sugars. It burns these sugars very rapidly creating a desire for more, and causing excessive oxidation resulting in an inflammatory response. This leads to obesity, premature aging, and a weakened immune system.

Natural sugars (occurring in whole fruits and vegetables) are part of a good nutritional package, have a lower GI, and are much healthier to eat. Eat foods with a low-GI such as beans, sweet potatoes, winter squashes and other vegetables, temperate fruits (berries, cherries, apples and pears) and less refined or processed food. While whole grain carbs are usually lower in GI, there is significant evidence out now that grains are just not good for us and should be very limited if eaten at all. Eating foods lower in GI will help avoid inflammation and blood sugar diseases as the body will process these foods in a more regulated manner.

The importance of good dietary fiber in our diets supports a healthy body and digestive system. Fiber is either *soluble* (coming from fruits, legumes, nuts, seeds, brown rice, oats, barley, and rice brans) or *insoluble* fiber (which comes from wheat and corn bran, whole grain breads and cereals, vegetables, fruit skins and nuts). Both are necessary but a good amount of insoluble fiber is important to healthy digestion and will alleviate digestive problems, especially in the colon. I have had clients with IBS and chronic diarrhea who have found huge relief just by adding a good fiber supplement (with no herbal laxatives) taken several times a day and eating digestive enzymes with meals. This step alone can be life changing.

Fats:

Fats are an important and necessary energy source. They carry certain nutrients and insulate our nerves and bones and provide essential nutrients for skin and hair. They are crucial for good brain health. But there are good fats and bad fats and it is important to choose your fats wisely. Saturated fats are primarily from meat sources. Most doctors agree that the amount of these fats should be somewhat limited; especially the ones found in red meats and processed foods. Mono-saturated and poly-unsaturated fats are the good fats found in olive oil, avocado oil and fish oils, and are known to lower cholesterol and aid in other body functions. **Beware of the commonly used vegetable oils, especially canola and palm oil, as these oils are not easily digested nor beneficial and are present in almost any foods you buy, even at health food stores.**

Choosing your fats wisely will help to balance your essential fatty acids and temper the inflammatory response in your body. Generally, the omega-6 fatty acids increase inflammatory reaction while the hormones we create from the omega-3 fatty acids cause a decrease of inflammation in the body. The Standard American Diet (SAD) is generally very high in omega-6. Vegetable oils are typically all high in omega-6 and low in omega-3. Fish oil supplements and foods including certain fish, flax seed, walnuts, and hemp are promoted now to build better health and even prevent heart disease and other chronic ailments. Most people should take an Omega-3 supplement containing a minimum of 1000 mg of EPA, DHA and other Omega 3's twice a day in addition to making good oil choices.

Vitamins:

Vitamins help to regulate chemical reactions in the body and are necessary for good health. There are 13 vitamins including Vitamins A, B's, C, D, E, and K. Because we cannot make vitamins in the body, they must be provided in our diet. There is a grand debate today as to whether vitamin supplements are necessary. I am of the opinion it is good for most people to take a high quality multi-vitamin *from a whole food source* and other supplements like fish oil as suited to one's individual needs. You can read more about supplements in Chapter 5.

Minerals:

Minerals are components of foods involved in many body functions. Calcium and magnesium are important for bone and digestive health. Iron is needed by our red blood cells to transport oxygen. There are primary minerals like calcium, magnesium, iron, and potassium and there are trace minerals like nickel and selenium that are needed by the body in only small amounts. Minerals will be discussed in Chapter 5 to help you decide if you are getting enough or should supplement.

Phytonutrients:

These are active organic compounds from fruits and vegetables that promote good health. They come in many classes, but you are may of heard of carotenoids, flavonoids, polyphenols and sulfides. The carotenoids give fruit and vegetables their red, orange, and yellow color and are believed to protect against certain cancers, heart disease, and vision loss. One orange contains over 170 phytonutrients. It is important to eat whole foods of varied colors daily if we want to add these critical nutrients to our diet. Think of a rainbow when you are preparing a meal. Try to prepare the most colorful dishes possible not only for visual appeal, but to give your family the widest range of phytonutrients possible.

In one study printed in the "Journal of the American Medical Association", consuming just three servings of fresh fruits and vegetables daily was linked to a 22% decreased risk of stroke. Overall, phytonutrients are believed to slow the aging process. Many protect against a host of illnesses and diseases (such as cancer, heart disease, and high blood pressure). They also enhance immunity and serve as antioxidants.

There are supplements that provide these nutrients too and many quality vitamins will have a phytonutrient base included to make the vitamins more available to the body.

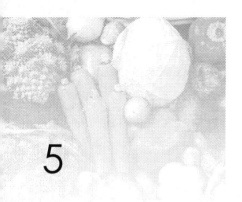

5

Proper Food Combining

▬ ▬ ▬ ▬ ▬ ▬

Incorrect food combining is one of the biggest problems with the Standard American Diet (SAD) - now spreading across the planet. This is the common meat and potatoes diet most of us were raised on. Hamburgers, turkey sandwiches or spaghetti and meatballs are good examples of what not to do in food combining.

Think of a hamburger comprised of a white bun and a hunk of meat, (the more meat the better, if you believe the ads.)

Often we gulp the food down on the run, entirely missing out on the first crucial step in breaking down the burger. Digestion begins in the mouth as our saliva combines with the food and starts to break it down. Saliva contains amylase, a digestive enzyme that begins to turn complex carbohydrates into simple carbohydrates. Most of us don't properly chew our food.

The smaller the food pieces entering the stomach, the more surface contact they get with the acids and enzymes that actually digest what we eat. Many nutritionalists believe that every mouthful should be chewed a very minimum of forty times. Try counting your chews the next time you eat or simply put your fork down between bites. It will slow you down. *Let your teeth do the work for your gut, unless you want a fat gut.*

As we chew the sandwich, it passes through the esophagus and into our stomachs where a highly acidic environment will attempt to break down and digest the proteins. Stomach secretions of gastric acid, largely comprised of hydrochloric acid, provide an acid environment with a pH of 1.5 to 3.5. These acids activate the digestive enzymes that attack the meat in the burger. Unfortunately, in our case, the stomach acids are quickly absorbed by the big bun surrounding it, causing the stomach to secret *more* acid.

The body is never able to properly digest the huge quarter pound of beef and the whole mess is then dropped into the intestinal tract to continue the digestive process. At this point, the food should be in a liquid or paste form. However, if digestion does not occur properly, the food will not be sufficiently broken down and commonly acid reflux disease results from too much acid secretion. This can lead to esophageal cancer if it continues for too long a time period.

The intestines are designed for the digestion of carbohydrates (the bun), the breakdown of fats and assimilation of the nutrients from the food. This requires the opposite pH and the body releases bile, made by the liver and secreted by the gall bladder, to raise the pH to the alkaline environment required in the intestines. Powerful enzymes secreted by the pancreas also play an important role here in the digestive process. With our hamburger, it is difficult to maintain the right pH environment because the wad of undigested meat and acid soaked bun neutralize the alkalinity preventing proper digestion from occurring. But the body tries its best. As you can see, we don't make it easy.

The small intestine is the site of the remaining digestion, through peristaltic movement and chemical reactions. In the healthy body, most absorption also takes place in the walls of the small intestine, which is densely folded to maximize the surface area in contact with digested food. Small blood vessels in the intestinal wall pick up the molecules after they are broken down and carry them to the rest of the body. If the food is not properly broken down at this stage of the digestive process, problems occur.

When the remaining food is dumped into the large intestine or colon, it contains water it has adsorbed as well as some remaining nutrients. Adequate levels of friendly bacteria are required in the colon for these functions to occur. That is why healthy probiotic balance and abundance are critical. If the balance of bacteria in the colon is disrupted, more digestive issues will arise. The large intestine plays a crucial role in a healthy digestive system as it deals with the waste that remains, preparing it to become feces and properly eliminated.

Compounding the digestive problems with meat and carbohydrate meals is the addition of sugar. That processed bun becomes pure sugar quickly in the gut and sugar causes fermentation or the formation of gas. This is made worse by the sugars that are added for "better" flavor to most foods. That is why so many people suffer from gas and bloating after eating. The intestines, like the stomach, cannot do an adequate job of digestion with this toxic bomb we have dumped into it. Undigested waste products fill the gut and incomplete elimination through the bowels leaves behind a host of substances that the body then needs to deal with. No wonder we feel tired or in need of a nap after a big meal with improper food combining. No wonder there are so many people who suffer from digestive problems. Our digestive systems are complex and well-designed, but only if we eat the right combinations of food to make food our friend.

Ever notice how some foods cause you to have horrible breath or that some dogs are prone to terrible smelling breath? This is an indication of poor digestion and can be remedied by proper food combining and adding digestive enzymes.

So how do we combine foods? To make it as easy as possible for our bodies to digest and utilize the nutrients in foods, the short answer is to eat very simply, not combining foods that require opposite acid/base environments in order to be digested i.e. the hamburger!

If you look back at how our earliest ancestors ate, the hunter-gatherers ate one type of food at a time. They ate the simple foods they could find or hunt as they found them. That is really how our bodies and our digestive systems are designed. Think of how good you feel when you eat a handful of fresh berries or a simple salad. Your body functions as it should and you are energized and feel light. As we add more foods to the mix, the body slows down and struggles to make anything digest well.

The worst combination possible is meat and carbohydrates, in other words the Standard American Diet (SAD). This is especially true for refined carbohydrates that quickly break down into sugars (white potatoes, white bread, and white rice) and red meats that are the hardest for our bodies to digest. If the *only* dietary change you make is to eat avoiding this combination, your life will change dramatically guaranteed. Improper digestion leads to chronic disease. It is the accumulation of toxic waste products in the cells and the lack of nutrient assimilation that leads to aging.

Digestive enzymes play a critical role in digestion and it is advised that you add a good digestive enzyme supplement to all of your meals. As we age, our bodies do not produce as many digestive enzymes as we need. Cooked and processed foods are devoid of live enzymes. If we do not supplement them, our bodies will steal pancreatic (also known as metabolic) enzymes normally needed for other body functions to help digest our food.

Protein molecules that are not fully digested in the stomach and colon are absorbed into the blood stream. Once in the bloodstream, the immune system treats them as invaders provoking an immune reaction. When these substances accumulate to the point that the lymphatic system cannot adequately deal with them, we see "allergic" reactions. As these foreign substances from inadequately digested food invade the body's soft tissues, inflammation develops. Inflammation is a major cause of most chronic disease. Take digestive enzymes with your meals and if possible, support your body with metabolic enzyme supplements to decrease inflammation and support all cellular activity. These enzymes are the ones taken between meals that your doctor or naturopath may prescribe for inflammatory conditions of all kinds. There are over 1000 enzymes in the human cell. Life cannot exist without them. Most of us are critically low on both types of enzymes in our bodies.

A full glass of water and a digestive enzyme 20 minutes to a half hour before lunch and dinner is highly beneficial. **Never ever drink water with your meals**. It dilutes the acids and bases needed for digestion in the gut and makes it even harder for the body to digest food. Water a half hour before a meal is a great habit to establish. You will find you eat less too as an added benefit. How we drink our water, in addition to getting proper quantities of healthy, chemical-free water, is crucial for a healthy digestive and metabolic system.

The first step in getting your body's digestive system working well is to do the 10-day Reboot Program which requires limits on carbs and never combines refined carbohydrates (like bread or pasta) with a complex protein like meat. Meals consist of lots of veggies with enough protein to provide nourishment. Usually fish or poultry are preferable to red meats. However, occasional red meat, especially grass fed beef or wild meats, may be beneficial for some people. Whole grain products are substituted for white ones if consumed at all and if you do eat a potato, it is a sweet potato. If you are vegetarian, it is more challenging to get sufficient and proper protein combinations, but it is possible and there will be a radical improvement in your health.

For optimal health and energy, a serving of fruit first thing in the morning followed by a protein based meal about a half an hour later is ideal. Follow with a complex carbohydrate either for a snack or lunch. This could be a slice of whole grain bread or a serving of oatmeal if you need it. (It is better to avoid all grains.) Your body will tell you when you need the carbohydrate, as you may feel slightly dizzy without some carbs by mid-morning depending on your body's blood sugar levels. Lunch is generally a salad with small amount of chicken or fish. An afternoon snack is a handful of nuts or veggies and dip (or nut butter) or a green drink. A typical dinner is chicken or fish (or veggie protein) and two servings of veggies. Another snack may be eaten around 7-8 p.m. and you are set for the day.

The rule for food combining is carbohydrates (like rice, potatoes, and bread) should only be eaten with veggies. For example, eat a veggie dish with whole grain pasta for lunch or a sandwich with veggies only, no meat. Complex proteins should only be eaten with veggies, preferably ones with low starch or carbs. In other words, keep the carbs and proteins as separate as possible. Nuts and fruits should be eaten alone to allow the body to digest and utilize their nutrients fully.

There are mixed nutrients in most foods, so many veggies contain both carbs and proteins. Don't be confused by this. The idea is to keep the starchy carbs and complex, hard-to-digest proteins separate in order to make digestion easier and to achieve good nutrient assimilation.

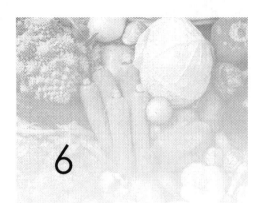

6

Vitamins and Supplements, to Do or Not to Do

The airwaves continue to offer up a multitude of negatives and cautions about vitamins and supplements. Some are founded, some are not. It is important to realize that a healthy nation is a huge threat to the medical and health care industry. Their business and profits come from our illnesses.

As a pharmacist, I find it sad that the American government allows TV ads for medications that must be prescribed by a doctor. This is a recent development allowing broad marketing of prescriptions to the public who have little knowledge regarding these drugs, only seeing pretty ads of what life could be like with the medication they are promoting. Many billions are spent each year on ads to encourage people to go see their doctor and request specific drugs. "Got an illness, we've got a cure," seems to be the attitude. They are not offering cures, treating only symptoms, not the cause of illness. It is a national disgrace that oncology physicians make money on chemotherapy drugs they prescribe. This makes the most expensive therapies more attractive as income generators and the advertising by the drug industry makes the cost of prescription drugs higher. But back to supplements…

Taking supplements should be an informed choice you make based upon real possible benefits to your health and vitality. Finding medical practitioners who are informed on supplements and can offer real advice can be challenging. Vitamins too are a huge industry and most people are wasting their money on things they don't need, sub therapeutic dosages of supplements or in some cases, things that can harm or create imbalance in the body. Be cautious of anyone who wants to sell you supplements as part of their practice or at least know that you may be paying a premium and many health care providers who make recommendations are not fully knowledgeable of *all* nutrients needed and may only "prescribe" ones for your symptoms.

It is important that any vitamins and supplements you take come from a reputable quality company. You may want to order your vitamins online to secure the freshest products and assure quality control. Some drug store varieties are synthetic vitamins that are manufactured from petrochemicals, and while their chemical structure may be identical, the benefits may not. It is highly probable that the vitamins in the products may not be as bioavailable (easily absorbed) as ones from natural food sources. We hear government recommendations to get your vitamins and minerals from your food, but the reality is most people do not eat enough fruits and vegetables to get sufficient vitamins. In addition, the foods we buy today in the grocery do not contain the same amounts of vitamins and minerals that foods used to because of severe soil depletion. This is well documented. Soils must be alive in order to grow nutritious food. Healthy soils are full of enzymes, microorganisms and micronutrients from plant and manure decomposition. Our foods are grown in an environment with pumped up nutrition, largely from chemical nitrogen fertilizers. A vegetable may sit in storage for weeks or even months before making it to your table, all the while the quality of nutrients offered deteriorates. If you only buy local organically grown food you *may* be getting more of what you need from your food. However, most of us do not.

To make matters worse, the environment contains many more toxic compounds than ever before. We have synthesized tens of thousands of new chemicals that the population was not exposed to in your parents' upbringing. Chemicals are everywhere including pesticides, herbicides, chemicals to flavor our food, and keep the foods, lotions and shampoos we use preserved or stable for long shelf lives. We are constantly bombarded by these chemicals and many have not been tested for toxic effects on humans. Antioxidants help to protect us from our environment; just as in nature, they protect the plant from injury. Many, like grape seed extract or pine tree bark extract (Pycnogenol) are found in the skin or outermost layer of the plant. Often when we eat plants, we peel off the skin and throw away the important vitamins and nutrients it contains.

In recent years, most doctors have come around to recommend a few supplements including fish oil, possibly Vitamin C, D and E or calcium. Some recommend a good multivitamin. Many recommend fiber as a supplement like the psyllium seed in Metamucil. Times have changed somewhat with greater acceptance by mainstream doctors of the need to supplement, but the fear campaign against supplements continues. Recently, there were studies publicized that showed possible increase in heart disease in women who took calcium supplements. The problem is that "scientific studies" are easily manipulated and can be used to make a point or wage a campaign so it is hard to know whom to believe.

A valid scientific study must have at least 600 participants, have double blind studies and be carefully planned and supervised by a neutral party to present a truly neutral outcome we can believe as true. Drug companies and university studies sponsored by drug companies are the biggest producers of studies. It must be in someone's interest to carry out a scientific study and generally, there is a desired outcome, which immediately invalidates the neutrality of the study.

Use some common sense and consider the following list of supplements as a baseline if you want optimal health. If you are treating a specific disease or dietary need, it is advisable to take supplements only under the supervision of a health care specialist, preferably one who has good knowledge of supplemental therapies.

Basic vitamins to consider adding to your diet:
1) **Antioxidants** like Vitamin C and E, grape seed extract, or pine tree bark are crucial as are anti-inflammatories like a high quality curcumin from turmeric. It is important

to take a bio-available curcumin if you chose to add this to your diet. While all multiples have some antioxidants in them, the amounts of these precious compounds from nature are probably not enough in a multiple for adequate protection from aging and disease.

2) A **multivitamin** from a whole food source with minerals is good for most people. (If your vitamin does not have minerals, you may want to add a multi-mineral supplement.) Many people are also deficient in **Vitamin D** so testing of Vitamin D levels is important as is getting a therapeutic dose from the supplement you take. Current recommendations are 10,000 i.u. per day unless you spend a lot of time in the sun. B vitamins are sometimes useful if you suffer from anemia or low energy. If you do take B's, chose a whole food source and take folate not folic acid as it is the form found naturally in the body.

3) **Calcium and magnesium** in a form that your body can assimilate is also important. Magnesium is often very useful for leg cramps as calcium/magnesium balance in our bodies is involved in muscle contractions. Calcium carbonate is not easily digested or utilized by the body, but it is the most common form of calcium found in supplements. This is because it is the least expensive. For example, antacids such as Tums are not a good source of calcium. If your doctor recommends them, I would consider changing doctors. Calcium and magnesium are vital for almost all cells and are crucial for good colon health and regular bowel movements. Most people

notice a difference in their bowels when they use these supplements, often noticing more bowel movements daily and lighter, fluffier feces. One way you can judge if your calcium and magnesium are being absorbed is if your bowel movements change for the better.

Many natural doctors and health practitioners believe that you should have a bowel movement for every meal you eat. I believe three to be the average for optimal health, but everyone is different and your bowel function may differ. There is an absolute need for a minimum of one bowel movement per day, preferably more. If you are not experiencing this, try adding calcium, magnesium, digestive enzymes and colon cleanser or fiber drinks. This is how we dispose of waste from our cells. Waste accumulation is toxic for health. *Health starts in the intestine and colon health is an overall health indicator.*

4) If you suffer from low energy or hair or skin and nail problems, you may want to consider a good **trace mineral supplement**. Unlike the minerals found in many multiples, trace minerals are taken in vary low doses. They provide critical roles in the body and are necessary for many enzyme and chemical reactions we depend on for good health.

5) **Digestive Enzymes** are needed by everyone over the age of 15 unless perhaps your diet consists of primarily raw vegetables and fruit or raw juices. Supplementation is the only way to get adequate enzymes. They help us to digest foods better and aid in nutrient assimilation. (If you have

taken antibiotics, digestive enzymes and probiotics are essential in rebuilding proper digestive health.)

6) **Fiber or colon cleansers** should be taken by all adults. We do not eat sufficient fiber in most of our diets to fulfill our needs. It is easy to take a psyllium based product in a morning shake if you have problems remembering to take supplements. Adding a colon cleanser in the morning and at night will make a huge improvement of digestive health for most people.

7) **Fish Oil or another source of Omega 3's and CoQ10 is another supplement to consider.** It is important that the supplement taken be mostly Omega 3's as the optimal balance of Omega 3's to Omega 6's in our diet is 2:1 and the average diet already contains significant amounts of Omega 6's. CoQ10 is recommended for most adults over the age of 30, as it declines in the body with age and offers good support for the heart and gum health in valid scientific studies.

8) Other supplements can be added to support various weaknesses on an individual basis. MSM, hyaluronic acid, glucosamine, and niacinamide are some that can greatly benefit our aging bones, joints, and skin. Some supplements support healthy blood sugar levels. There are good supplements to supplement our brain nutrients and help balance our moods instead of antidepressants or other drugs. Others supplements support immune disfunction or other disease states. If you are a vegetarian,

you will want to supplement with vitamin B12 and B6 and possibly zinc and calcium.

It is important to know that what you are taking is safe. Carefully research or rely on a knowledgeable health professional to guide you. Some supplements can have toxic effects if taken in excess, so it is important to be smart about your choices.

A healthy diet consisting of lots of water, fruit and vegetables and mostly natural foods provides the best framework for all of us to begin. Remember your food is still more important than any supplements. If you eat poorly, all the supplements in the world will not provide you with good health. That said, I take a lot of supplements and feel it well worth the investment in my health. Working with a good functional medicine doctor or nutritional coach can help you to learn what supplements are most appropriate for you.

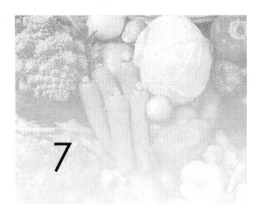

7

Making Mealtime Special Again

▄▄ ▄▄ ▄▄ ▄▄ ▄▄ ▄▄

In today's world approximately half of our meals are eaten away from home and most on the run. It is crucial to make an effort to reclaim the family meal time ritual that every culture and nationality seems to have in their heritage. Eating dinner watching TV is not mindful eating. So, how do we re-establish this custom?

With intent and follow-through. We must commit to doing it. The rest is easy.

At least one or more meals a day should be eaten with family or those you live with. If you live alone, at least once a day, take the time to sit at a table and simply eat with intention and enjoyment of the meal.

When our daughter was growing up, often the only time the family came together and truly shared an eating experience was dinner. Yes, there would be the nights when after basketball or soccer, we would go have pizza, but even then we would always try to sit and eat together, enjoying the food and each other's company.

Guidelines for Intentional Eating:

- Plan ahead. It makes life much easier and you will eat more healthy nourishing food if you plan meals ahead of time. It takes the stress out of "What's for dinner?" and trying to find something to eat after a busy day. I suggest a week at a time or at least 3-4 days, whatever fits with your shopping schedule. (You will also save money as the broccoli hiding in the back of the veggie bin has a specific date with the skillet or pan.)

- Stop the clock, take time to lovingly prepare what it is you are going to eat, even if it is a five minute prep time meal. Some people enjoy pouring a glass of wine or flavored sparkling water for themselves or putting on an apron or music as they start to work. Whatever you enjoy that makes the prep time more of a ritual, and signifies something important is about to happen, works and is important, setting the stage for an enjoyable meal.

- Prepare the eating area for the meal. Set the table carefully paying attention to detail whether it is folding napkins or putting them into napkin rings. Do it with joy, creating a peaceful, relaxing environment. Flowers or candles and a table free of clutter add to an enjoyable experience. Because we always had flowers or candles at the dinner table, so does my daughter. It is a custom worth passing on.

- Insist that when the meal is ready, all family members come at once and **leave their phones and electronic devices away**

from the table. Turn the TV off. Nothing is more important than this time together and interruptions of texting or phones answered need to be prohibited. It can always wait until after the meal.

- Take a moment when everyone (or just you if eating alone) sits down to pause from your busy day and be grateful for the food. This does not have to be a religious moment, just a time to feel a sense of gratitude and take a breath together. Maybe look each person at the table in the eye and really connect. Some find saying grace together the best way to accomplish this. It is up to you to honor the moment, connect and be grateful.

- Bring back the manners. Napkins on the laps, passing dishes to each other, taking time to ask the others how their day was. This is a time to connect not only with the food but also with each other.

- Eat slowly, chewing each bite more than you normally would and really *taste* the food. Notice what you like or love and what you aren't really impressed with. Try to find something you like in foods you may not normally eat and try them all, even if they are not something you normally eat. Remember it is polite to eat what you are served with respect and honor for the person or people who worked to prepare it and gratitude for the plants and animals that gave their lives so you could eat this food before you.

- Everyone sits at the table until all are finished eating at our house. There is no jumping up to run back to the internet or TV or even to start the dishes. This is respectful to all.

- Eating a meal is a sacred time. Take your time and enjoy this time together, or if you are by yourself, enjoy your own company and what you have laid out before you, practicing mindfulness and intentional eating with every bite.

- When the last person finishes, leave the table together, helping to clear the table and sharing in the clean-up. An exception to this may be a situation where the person preparing the meals may rely on the rest of the family to do cleanup without them. That works well as long as the mealtime tasks are shared!

- Even the dish washing and clean up is part of this special time and can be done with love and mindfulness. Enjoy it!

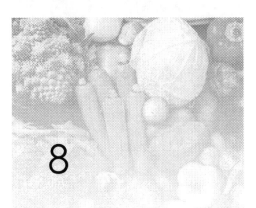

8

How to Shop, What to Buy

▬ ▬ ▬ ▬ ▬ ▬

Remember, the quality of the food is more important than what you eat. Buy the freshest food you possibly can is crucial to healthy eating, or better yet, grow it yourself. You want to value your food enough to take the time to seek out or grow the best you can.

If you have a local farmer's market, this is the place to start your food shopping. Buying locally grown food from the person who grew it is the next best thing to growing it yourself. Try to buy as much as you can at the market, remembering to check the food inventory at home before you go so as not to buy what is already in the fridge and needs to be used.

Shopping starts at home. Make a list of what you need based on what you have on hand and what you plan to cook. Write up your menu and keep a list going throughout the week in a place where all family members can add to it if something they like to eat is needed.

When you are at the market or even the grocery, take your time and enjoy the shopping process. Don't shop when you are hungry or when you are in a hurry. Schedule time to do it right. Talk to the people you meet and the employees you encounter. It matters and makes the shopping experience a special time. Shopping is personal. I enjoy complimenting people in a chain produce department if I find a great selection of fresh organic produce. Ask questions to learn more about the food you are buying.

Now you have your list and you have scheduled the time. It can be a family event or you can shop alone. Either way -- enjoy it.

In a traditional grocery store, the place to shop is the very outside edge of the store. That is where you will find the fresh food that will nourish you and your family. I like starting in produce. I like the colorful displays and take time to observe and enjoy them. Let the fruits and veggies call out to you, energetically speaking.

As you circle around the store, you will find the meats, fish, and then dairy. If your cart is already full, you will not need a lot here, maybe just some kefir or Greek yogurt (no added sugars please). Use cheese if you eat it, as a seasoning, not a staple.

Skip the bakery and deli unless you perhaps wish some olives from the olive bar or other food that is real and something you can use in your planned meals. If you must buy bread, make sure it is whole grain (sprouted if possible) or gluten-free if you prefer. It is better to use alternative grains to wheat and to eat as few grains as possible.

Find the bulk foods section, if you are lucky enough to have one in your store. Stock up on nuts and seeds as well as spices and herbs that are fresh and make your food more interesting and tasteful.

Now, it is time to leave. Avoid the freezer and refrigerator sections, the prepared food aisles and all the packaged goods and sweets. You will save time and money by becoming a more *mindful* shopper. If you must buy veggies that are processed, frozen is much more nutritious than canned.

Be thankful and proud of yourself for a successful trip to the store. Smile as you walk or drive away.

Basic Foods to Have in Your Pantry & Refrigerator:

Oils: olive oil (for cooking), Extra Virgin olive oil (for salads and low temperature cooking only), coconut oil, avocado oil (both good for hi temps), pure sesame oil for seasoning. You just cannot find prepared salad dressings that are healthy and free of bad oils. Read the labels; you are likely to find canola or vegetable oils even if it says 'Olive Oil' on the front label. Preferably make your own salad dressings. Even if you use a flavoring packet, you can use good healthy oils and vinegars.

Condiments: ginger root, turmeric, dried basil, rosemary, thyme, garlic (fresh & granulated), any other dried herbs you like to cook with, Dijon mustard, heathy mayonnaise salad dressing, homemade or healthy ranch dressing, balsamic vinegar, sea salt, pepper, chili pepper flakes, dried peppers (if you like it hot).

Dried Goods: brown rice, quinoa, quinoa and brown rice pasta, dried beans and lentils (or canned), stock (low sodium chicken or veggie or make your own), coconut water, unsweetened milk substitute (almond, rice, soy, oat, hemp), nuts (preferably raw, unsalted), dried shredded coconut (optional), flaxseeds, chia seeds, (buy only seeds or nuts you will use), nutritional yeast (optional flavoring agent), spirulina or green powders (optional), protein powder of your choice. Mixed plant based or bone broth proteins are healthier than soy or whey. Read the label for hidden sugars.

Refrigerated & Fresh: lots of veggies (your choice for salads, green drinks, dinner sides like sweet potatoes), fruits (try to stick to lower sugar varieties like apples, berries, cherries and eat no more than two servings a day early in the day), local or organic eggs, plain kefir or plain or Greek yogurt, coconut milk, fresh salsa, guacamole, hummus, lemons, limes, nut butters, sparkling water, bottled seasonings like low sodium soy sauce, tamari or Braggs Liquid Aminos, quality peanut sauce, Szechwan sauce, chili sauce, fish sauce. Avoid any products with MSG, nitrates or other preservatives, added sugars, or hidden glutens.

Frozen: frozen berries for smoothies and quick special treats, chopped spinach, stir-fry mix (if you don't want to cut up your own), frozen kale cubes for homemade smoothies. It is always better to cut up and make your own frozen fruits and vegetables for smoothies but if necessary, buy prepackaged organic ones in store.

9

Basic Skills of Cooking

▬ ▬ ▬ ▬ ▬ ▬

Tools:

Whether cooking in a lovely kitchen with lots of amenities and space, or an RV or around a campfire, it is important to have the right tools. Your living environment and your time to spend preparing food are considerations that will determine what you need for tools. Below I deal with the basics to do it well.

You need good knives for trimming, chopping and cutting through foods you plan to cook. You need a range of pots, pans, and strainers that meet your needs well and are healthy to use. I recommend the new ceramic pans and skillets available but stainless and other healthy alternatives also are good. Avoid Teflon and aluminum.

Other kitchen supplies could include measuring implements, colanders, spatulas, cooking spoons, glass or other healthy material casserole dishes or baking pans, and anything else you need for the preparation.

The right tools make it easier. Even when I am in the RV traveling, I carry my food processor and juicer. The one appliance that I believe is a must for everyone is a juicer of some sort. Green drinks are a part of healthy living today and a medicine all of us need. To make it easiest to use and clean, I prefer the ease of a NutriBullet but a good blender or high-end juicer is fine as long as it can liquefy vegetables like kale, carrots, etc. Something that facilitates quick use and easy cleanup can be easily incorporated into your mealtime routines. Juicers that extract the pulp are time consuming to clean so unless you really dislike the pulp, leave it in using a blender style juicer and save yourself a lot of time.

Style:

OK, you are ready to go. You have the foods. You have the right tools. Now, what are you going to make with them? That is up to you. We all have different likes and are limited by the amount of time we have to spend in the kitchen. How elaborate or simple do you want to go? Are you drawn by the "simple, quick dinners for people on the go" headlines on magazines and cookbooks or the more elaborate and time-consuming themes? This will determine your direction. Either way, I recommend spending some time to figure out what type of meals you want to prepare and write down some meal ideas that appeal to you. Good food does not have to be fancy and some of my best gourmet meals are the most simple to make. I generally look for recipes with the fewest ingredients for everyday meals.

Methods:

There are basic methods of cooking depending on what you are trying to accomplish. I am going through the basics below to encourage people with little or no cooking skills to give it a try.

Raw Food Preparation:

Most of us eat at least some raw foods if only in the way of carrot or celery sticks and salads. If you are eating primarily raw foods, cutting boards and knives will be important, saucepans not so much. Raw foods do require more thought and planning for balanced diets and a bigger area in the refrigerator if you do not have an active garden year round. You can find good cook books for smoothies and green drinks, wonderful salads and even uncooked healthy snacks. For example, wonderful snacks can be made from almond meal, coconut, chocolate ground together with a bit of oil and maybe adding some fresh blueberries before patting out into a pan and refrigerating to set. Ground cashews can make a nice alternative to cheese or yogurt and make lovely sauces. The possibilities are endless and lots of raw food recipes are available online. Soaking nuts overnight makes them more digestible.

Steaming:

Many believe that steaming is the best way to gently cook vegetables to preserve the most enzymes and nutrients. It requires some sort of steaming tray if you are to keep the veggies out of the water while they cook. Inexpensive steaming inserts can be found to make this easier. Steamed veggies can be combined with healthy oils, seasonings, and herbs and served with or without protein or carbohydrate main dishes. Don't overcook! Steamed veggies should still have a bit of crunch.

Stir-Fry:

This is the style of cooking I use most. With the wonderful variety of healthy oils now available, and the new way of thinking that good oils are good for your body, why not? Stir-fry can be Asian, Mediterranean or any other flavor you like. It's not just Chinese anymore! In late summer when my garden produces more tomatoes, beans and zucchinis more than broccoli, snow peas or bok choy, I make a stir-fry that uses these veggies. Chopped tomatoes are a wonderful and varied addition at the end to make a sauce. You can add things like olives, garbanzo beans, and fresh herbs like basil and oregano or dill or even chili sauce to create interesting dishes with short prep times. One of my summer "use those beans and zucchini" dishes starts with olive oil and lots of garlic, then either chopped green beans or zucchini scoops (from insides of a larger zucchini). Then simmer until done, simple and yummy. With the green beans, I add some chopped tomatoes and cook until the tomatoes make a creamy coating on the beans. This keeps well in fridge and can be enjoyed cold or warm. See recipes and resources for more ideas on how to cook easily and quickly this way with what you have in garden or fridge.

For a basic stir-fry, start with an oil that can handle higher heats, either avocado oil, coconut oil or a non-virgin olive oil. Heat oil in the pan, add any seasonings you wish like chopped garlic, ginger and/or green onions, stir a minute, then add the veggies that take the longest to cook. Stir-fry for a minute or so and add the next longest cooking veggies and continue until all veggies you want are in the pan and have had a quick toss around to heat thoroughly. If you are preparing a stir-fry with meat or fish, it is best to cook the meat first, remove from pan and set aside to add back to the dish right before serving. Meat should be thinly sliced or diced and you may want to marinate it with a mix of soy sauce and a bit of cornstarch or other thickener. Equal amounts of each work well with just enough to barely coat the meat.

At this point, you are ready to add some seasonings and liquid. You can drizzle with soy sauce, add a prepared sauce (be mindful of all the ingredients) like Peanut Sauce or Szechuan sauce, stir, then add a bit of stock or water and cover to briefly steam. (If you are doing a Mediterranean style stir-fry, add your chopped tomatoes if desired and cook with no lid on low until the desired consistency.) With a traditional stir-fry, you can add any final seasonings or a tiny bit of thickener if you wish, and serve.

Baking:

Almost anything can be baked. It is simple and can be useful for entertaining or a one dish family meal. Baking veggies gives them a unique and nice flavor, just don't overcook them. Always cook poultry to at least 160 degrees Fahrenheit. Veggies can be added to meat or poultry dishes part way through so as not to overcook. Almost any type of sauce or stock can be added, or you can bake veggies just misted with olive or coconut oil. Wonderful sweet potato fries can be made in the oven and baked beets are a common ingredient in the gourmet salad selection at many fine restaurants. In summer, I enjoy a simple baked veggie casserole made by coating cut veggies with olive oil and lots of chopped garlic, then adding some chopped tomatoes part way through the baking time. Baking takes more time and a bit more know how than simple steaming or stir-fry but can add some variation to your mealtimes and offer you more away from the kitchen time right before the meal.

To many, baking means cakes, cookies and breads and this is an area we need to show some restraint if we are to eat healthy. While you can substitute better flours for wheat flour and stevia for sugar, the very nature of baked pastries and bread is not something we want to focus our eating on. These baked goods should be saved for occasional treats and bread is better avoided or limited to early day consumption in moderation only.

Barbecuing or Grilling:

The new infrared barbecues offer a healthier way to grill meat as they avoid the charcoal grill that leaves the residue high in nitrates linked to causing cancer. As a rule, it is wise to avoid burned or dark cooked foods in general. Grilling is easy once you get to know your grill and a simple chicken breast can make an ultra simple meal combined with a salad and veggies. This type of cooking works well for some as a staple as it is something quick and easy that is also very healthy if done right. Don't forget to experiment with grilled veggies. They too love a marinade and keep the summertime kitchen cool. Try olive oil, garlic, and lemon, adding some fresh herbs of your choice.

Microwaving:

Yes, it is fast and works well with prepared foods. That is probably a good reason to avoid it. In addition, microwaving foods kills off the enzymes more than any other form of cooking and puts off microwaves that are not healthy to be within close proximity. I recommend not using a microwave unless you absolutely must and then doing as little as possible using it. If you meet someone that predominately uses a microwave for cooking, the chances are they won't be very healthy.

Broiling:

This is very similar to barbecuing as you are really using a heat source close to the meat or veggie to cook and heat it quickly with some browning. Again, avoid burning or over browning foods, as they are not healthy for you containing cancer producing chemicals.

Boiling or simmering:

Boiling or simmering works well with some foods that typically take longer to cook. This type of cooking would include the use of a slow cooker where all of the foods are added together and they cook for a number of hours. I often quickly parboil sweet potatoes before adding them to a dish with spinach in olive oil and garlic. (See recipe ideas section.) The only caution here is when foods are cooked with liquid in a boil or simmer and the liquid is discarded, many of the vitamins and nutrients are thrown out with the bath water. Also, there may be a tendency to overcook foods with a slow cooker or by boiling so remember the nutrients go way down when veggies are overcooked. The glycemic index also goes up making them harder on your body's attempts to keep a balanced blood sugar level.

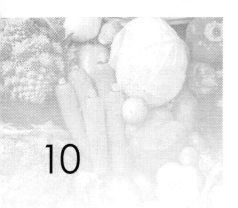

10

To Meat or Not to Meat

A major question all of us face is whether to eat meat or not. Some of you may be vegan or vegetarian, but meat is still a staple in the diet for most people.

In my more than twenty years of nutritional counseling, I have found that the basic truth is some people do better with some meat in their diet, whereas some are healthy and vital as vegetarians or vegans. I have come to believe that our genetic makeup and body type may have a role in determining if we need meat in our diet or can exist and flourish without it.

While there are many healthy vegetarians, it is very important to know that a strict vegetarian or vegan diet does pose health risks if you are not aware of methods to attain all of your basic nutrients using this type of diet. Vitamin D, Vitamin B12, zinc and calcium are some of the nutrients that are difficult to get in sufficient amounts. Vitamin B12 only occurs in meat products.

Additionally, vegetarians may be prone to eat food science products like phony ground meat, mock cheese, and dairy. While there are a few good products available in these categories, most contain more carbs, sugars, and other ingredients that may even be harmful to your health. Read the labels carefully before buying any of these products. You may be amazed at some of the ingredients you find in the "health food" section.

Often, vegetarians rely on carbs and may develop quite severe sugar addictions. Too many carbs from grains or unrefined carbs that quickly become sugars lead to weight gain or possible severe digestive disorders. Conversely, some vegetarians or vegans lose too much weight.

The consequences of poor decisions often made by vegetarians may be anemia, hypoglycemia, diabetes, dental problems, or osteoporosis. Even though one is less likely to have high blood pressure, high cholesterol, heart disease or type 2 diabetes as a vegetarian, you may be putting your health at risk unless you research what comprises a healthy vegetarian diet carefully.

Imagine eating a vegetarian diet, thinking you are eating healthy, only to have a tooth fall out unexpectedly from calcium deficiency and bone loss. This happened to the man who eventually founded the Vegetarian Health Institute. On the website for this organization, you can learn how to get the basic nutrition you need from grains and vegetables and basic food combining to optimize the absorption of vitamins and minerals from your foods. If you do choose to eat without meat and/or dairy, there are many other resources to learn how to eat well for optimal health including books and web information from nutrition experts like Dr. John McDougall, Dr. Michael Klaper, and Dr. Gabriel Cousins.

Other disadvantages of a meatless diet include the fact fresh vegetables are prone to lose their nutrients quickly after being harvested, spoiling rather quickly and they are expensive, especially if you buy local organic produce with the most nutrients in it. Many vegetarian recipes are time-consuming to prepare and call for uncommon and expensive ingredients. Packaged foods and restaurant meals often contain slaughterhouse by-products so careful vigilance in food choices is required to avoid hidden meat by-products. Also, sticking to a vegetarian diet may be difficult while traveling.

That said, a diet without meat can be very healthy, *more so* than one with meat. Meat is higher on the food chain. The lower on the food chain our food choices, the less likely we are to get toxic chemicals and other pollutants or hormones from our foods. These products, present in some amount in all foods, are much higher in meat and dairy than vegetables, nuts, seeds and grains.

Another benefit to a vegetarian diet is to the planet. Meat production uses more planetary resources and causes global warming. Many more people could be feed with the resources put into raising food today if it were all vegetable and grain based. The energy used in food production would be significantly lowered, as would be the damage to the environment.

Clearing and burning the rainforest in South America to raise cattle is an example of the planetary destruction caused by the meat industry. Huge amounts of resources and energy are used just to grow the grain just to feed the animals used in the meat industry. As the earth's population grows, the damaging impact of meat eating on the environment increases.

Many people are vegetarians because they are ethically opposed to the mass killing and inhumane treatment of the animals. Even the raising of eggs has become a huge industry with most chickens confined to small cages or crammed into spaces that would sicken the stomach of even the strongest amongst us. John Robbins makes a strong argument for giving up meat in his book <u>Diet for a New America</u>. I highly recommend reading it.

If you do choose to eat meat or dairy, it is important to source your meat and dairy products from local and humane sources. This may be difficult and expensive, often making organic local vegetables seem cheap in comparison. It is important to only consume whole mild dairy. The processing making dairy low fat or non fat makes the products very difficult to digest and the fat in the products is good for you, not something to be avoided. The mega-food industry is tricky in their labeling and terms too. A product can be labeled 'pasture raised' if the animal is exposed to five minutes of fresh air a day. A chicken can be labeled 'cage free' when it lives out its life in a crowded facility packed solid with other chickens or in only slightly larger cages. Pasture raised cows may be fed grains to fatten them before slaughter and that grain may be GMO corn or soy. The meat eater must learn to read labels and know the real difference in the terms used. To get quality products, freer from contaminants and toxins and humanely raised, he or she may spend significantly more money than the person buying regular meat products from the local grocery.

These are all considerations in choosing whether to eat meat or not. I believe that it must be a personal decision and there is no right or wrong. What is right for my body may not be what is right for you and what I believe about the ethics of eating meat or dairy may not be what you believe. Choose carefully and whatever your choice, do it with mindfulness and intention.

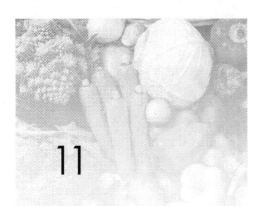

11

The Raw Foods Controversy

▬ ▬ ▬ ▬ ▬ ▬

Raw foods advocates tend to be adamant about the value of eating only raw foods because they believe raw foods contain enzymes and other nutrients that may break down during heating or cooking. These enzymes improve digestion and help the body absorb beneficial nutrients. Some people really thrive on a raw food diet, but others don't.

While the theory behind raw foods is plausible in many respects, it runs contrary to traditional Chinese and Ayurvedic teachings. These well-respected health systems state that nutrients from cooked food are more digestible because the cooking process breaks them down into smaller components, thereby supporting our "digestive fire" or a warmth and movement that brings vitality to the digestive tract and maintains our overall health. Chinese traditional wisdom is that light cooking or stir-frying makes foods more digestible.

An interesting fact to point out is that raw food diets tend to be more popular in warmer climates, such as Hawaii, Florida, and Southern California. This makes sense, as traditional Chinese medicine asserts that raw foods have a cooling effect on the body. Someone with a lot of inflammation, or heat, may find balance and greater vitality with a raw food diet. Conversely, someone who frequently feels cold can become weaker on a long-term raw food program.

Some nutrients become more bioavailable once they are heated. Lycopene, for example, an antioxidant found in tomatoes, carrots and other foods, is shown to be more nutritionally available when cooked. Vegetables such as kale, spinach, onions, and garlic are also shown to be more nutritious when cooked because light cooking releases compounds that might otherwise go undigested. Of course, overcooking foods, particularly meats, produces acrylamide and other chemicals that contribute to inflammation and cancer. As always, balance is important.

If you are considering starting a raw foods diet, I would suggest additional research on your part and trying it out to see how it affects your digestion and overall energy levels. For some people, raw foods are hard to digest. Others may not enjoy the somewhat limited types of dishes available or the work required to make raw foods meals varied and attractive.

Juicing is a raw foods preparation. Advocates of juicing believe that when you juice, foods are easier to digest since they are totally liquefied. This seems to be true and I am a strong advocate of juicing for at least one or two meals a day. I enjoy a protein shake in the morning and a green drink mid-afternoon so my juicer sees at least twice a day usage.

Raw foods eating is not all or nothing! Even if you do not want to commit to total raw foods as your diet, it is good to add raw veggies to your meals as much as you can, listening of course to your body and how well you digest them. Chewing becomes very important with raw foods to break them down as much as possible before they hit your digestive tract. I strongly advocate for a green drink in everyone's daily diet, just to increase your nutrients and crank up your energy levels in your body. Try juicing for nutrient supplementation -- you will like it.

A raw foods diet is not for everyone and if you decide to try it, listen to your body, and be sure to get enough Vitamin D and calcium, as bone health is a major concern both with raw food and vegan diets. In addition, it may be possible to lose your ability to eat and digest cooked foods over time, limiting what you can eat when you travel or are with people who do not eat raw foods.

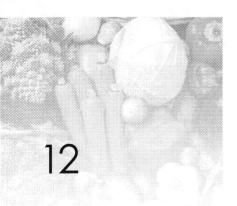

12

Everything in Moderation, Listen to Your Body

▬ ▬ ▬ ▬ ▬ ▬

The ultimate goal of this book is to assist you the reader in 1) breaking food addictions to sugar, salt and bad fats, 2) rebooting your metabolism to cleanse, purify and reset the naturally balanced systems in your body, 3) to assist you in identifying the right way of eating *for you* that will nourish and sustain your body to be its most healthy and vital self, and finally 4) to learn to eat with intention and awareness in every bite. I hope you are guided to find a way of eating that you love and is natural for you because it *feels* right.

The "feels right" part is so important because without learning to listen to your body, you can never get where you want to go. It is listening to that deep inner voice that will tell you, "Yes, I am full" or "No, that is too sweet for me!" Your body will tell you if it is happier on an all raw veggie diet, a vegan diet, a Paleo diet, or a way of eating that is your own creation. It will tell you if meat is something you need, how often you need it and what kind of meat to eat. But you can only discover these preferences when you learn to allow yourself to eat with awareness and intention. Your body knows, and every person has their own perfect diet. Take the time to learn to listen and you too will be able to eat what your body needs and benefits most from. It's time to live a lifestyle that does not involve restriction, labeling, or putting yourself in a box.

Remember quality is the most important factor that runs though any type of eating. Buy or grow the best food you can and eat regularly at least five times a day. Make healthy plant-based food your foundation from which to expand and explore. Eat well, eat clean, eat what you like because it nourishes your body and makes you feel good!

You may still have an occasional craving for an old 'baddie' or even have periods where you don't eat well for awhile, BUT… hopefully; those times will be short lived, if they occur at all. Just don't lose the truths you have discovered on our journey together about what good food is and what foods your body needs to be energetic, healthy and vital. Good healthy eating is a habit and it takes time and commitment to fully establish a good relationship with food. Then the right foods *for you* are a delight and easy to enjoy.

I hope you are now committed to undertake this courageous journey of self-discovery and allowing your body to heal by giving it what it needs. Remember, "Our body is the perfect healer," and "All healing is self-healing." I encourage you to work with a functional medical professional or a wellness coach, especially if you suffer from a serious or chronic disease. Changing your diet may upset your blood sugar level if you are diabetic or affect prescription medications so radical changes should be supervised and monitored if you have a chronic condition. A good functional medicine doctor or other practitioner knowledgeable in alternative healing will guide you in making the right choices about nutrition and supplements, as well as provide you with the support you need when you need it most. The more unbalanced your eating habits, the more you need to change them quickly. However, to embark upon this journey means only *when you are ready*. This is important and your first lesson in listening to your body. As Diane McLaren says,

"Within each of us, nature has provided all the pieces necessary to achieve exceptional health and wellness, then left it up to us to put them all together." Listen…

To conclude, may your food be your medicine. Be well and thrive. Enjoy every mouthful of good, healthy food with mindfulness and intention. Remember that *Intention* and *Attention* are the moment-to-moment principles to guide you to your strongest, most energized, healthy and vital self.

> **"Take care of your body. It is the only place you have to live."**
>
> **— Jim Rohn**

APPENDIX A: REBOOT PROGRAM GUIDE
10 (or 21 Day) Cleanse & Metabolism Reboot

Prohibited Foods:
- All Dairy (yes, that means cheese) except plain unsweetened yogurt or kefir
- All Fruit Juices and Fresh Fruit (except small serving blueberries or other fruit in morning smoothie or on oatmeal)
- Dried Fruit
- Sugar and Artificial Sweeteners
- Protein Bars
- White Potatoes
- Rice
- Pasta
- Bread
- Crackers
- Cookies, Muffins, Baked Goods.
- Cereals (except non-instant oatmeal)
- Other Processed Foods (canned soups, salad dressings, condiments, etc.)
- Alcohol
- Pop or Diet Soda
- Candy including Chocolate
- All Oils **EXCEPT** Olive, Coconut, Avocado Oil, Flax or Sesame Oil. (Eat as much of the good oils as you can!!)
- Coffee (see note below)

Helpful Hints:

There are two supplements I strongly advise people to use during the cleanse:

1) Start each day with a **fiber or colon cleanse**, preferably psyllium based, mixed in water followed by a full glass of water, then have the same colon cleanser before bed.

2) The second one is a good **digestive enzyme** that you take 20 minutes before eating your main meals (lunch and dinner). We are all lacking in enzymes from our food and this allows cleansing and getting maximum nutrition from your food.

Plan ahead. Have cut up veggies and other snacks ready and something with you at all times for snacks.

Have veggies cleaned and ready to snack on, add to salads or juice (making it almost effortless to whip up a green drink).

Read labels for hidden sugars in salad dressings, ketchup, seasonings, etc. The more you can get the bad foods out of your kitchen before starting, the better.

When shopping at grocery store, avoid processed foods entirely, shopping on outer edge of store only for fresh veggies, fruits, meats, fish and herbs. (Some seasonings may be OK but read the labels carefully).

Coffee is better skipped but if you need your cup, limit it to one, (no dairy or creamer). It is preferable to substitute green and herbal teas.

SO WHAT CAN I EAT? SOME SUGGESTIONS

Breakfast

Protein shake with 1/4 cup frozen fruit, kefir or yogurt (if you like), protein powder or nuts, seeds and other protein sources, green supplement if desired, coconut or flax oil (1 TBL) **OR** Eggs with vegetables

OR 1/2 c oatmeal with small amount of fruit (**avoid all carbs** for maximum weight loss, eat it if your body needs some carbs for blood sugar, i.e. if you feel dizzy or weak)

Snacks

-Oatmeal if you need it and did not have it earlier (Better as morning snack than for breakfast)

-Hard boiled or deviled egg

-Pickles

-Small handful of nuts, raw and unsalted

-Almond, peanut or cashew nut butter by itself or with celery

-Vegetables with hummous dip or guacamole

Lunch

-Salad with protein, veggie or chicken or fish broiled or steamed (Olive oil and vinegar or olive oil and lime based dressing.)

-Avocado stuffed with shrimp, tuna, chicken or veggie protein

-Turkey or baked chicken salad wrap (or fish) in lettuce with veggies. (Watch the condiments to avoid sugars!)

Snack -same ideas as above **OR** Green **OR** Red veggie drink (see recipes in Appendix B)

Dinner

    -Broiled or baked chicken or fish with two vegetables or one vegetable and a salad. Sweet potatoes OK as one vegetable but not every day.

    -Vegetarians and vegans eat a salad or multiple veggies with no added carbohydrates, focusing on proteins and greens.

Evening Snack (Same ideas as above but smaller quantities and at least 1-2 hrs. before bed)

WATER SCHEDULE FOR HEALTHY LIVING

-Drink lots of water! Carry it with you always.

-Drink one full glass on arising

-Drink one full glass a half hour before each meal and often throughout day between meals and on the go

-Drink one glass at bedtime and have a glass beside your bed stand to sip on if you wake up in night

DO NOT DRINK WATER OR ANY OTHER BEVERAGES <u>WITH YOUR MEALS</u>!!! (Liquids with meals dilutes stomach acid causing your body to secret more, iced cold solidifies bad fats into undigestible form, inhibits proper digestion...)

APPENDIX B:
SMOOTHIE & JUICING BASIC RECIPES

Basic ingredients: (adjust to your tastes but do try new foods too!)

Organic apples (I prefer green)

Kale (Red Russian is milder than the green)

Other hearty greens such as beet greens, Swiss chard, collard greens

Carrots

Celery

Cucumber

Any other greens or veggies on hand

Cooked or raw beets

Ginger root (use about 1/2 inch piece to taste)

Tumeric root (optional, great for inflammation and chronic pain)

Kombucha (optional, added at end for flavor and alkalinity)

Coconut water or filtered water and a few ice cubes

These are the primary veggies I use, but you can use any in your refrig too and experiment with new ones. Great way to never throw veggies away again, even leftover salad! Try small amounts of cabbage, cauliflower, broccoli, beans, whatever, ...You can even put tomatoes with veggies and make your own V8 juice (with hot sauce?) If you keep amounts small, nothing will be overpowering. It is always preferably to buy organic if possible.

If you are using a NutraBullit, the instructions say add water to the line on blender cup (NEVER OVERFILL) after you put in chopped up veggies and fruit. I like using at least half something other than water with more flavor and nutrients, i.e. bit of unsweetened cranberry juice, a splash of kombucha, or coconut water. If you are using a conventional juicer that removes the pulp, the extracted juices will be more concentrated and you do not need to add any additional liquids.

I prepare the veggies when I bring them home from the store or pick them from the garden, so it is really easy to make the smoothies in five minutes from start through cleanup. With kale, you cut off biggest part of stem, wash and chop coarsely, then bag. Carrots and celery, wash and cut into sticks in baggie (or use small organic carrots in bag). You can pre-wash the apples, cucumbers, broccoli, cauliflower or whatever else you choose. If it is pre-washed and bagged, it makes it very easy to throw a half handful in your smoothie.

To make a smoothie, use only the larger size mixer container of the NutraBullit. It makes a large glass serving that would probably be plenty for two starting out with a green drink. Go slowly with the green and red drinks as they are potent and may upset your stomach or cause diarrhea in some people not used to them.

Basically, I like to do a few basic smoothies and vary it by what is in refrig, but you can play with ingredients too and look for other recipes online. Look in the resource chapter for some easy online sources.

Fruit Protein Smoothie (morning meal or morning snack)

Handful of frozen berries (I like blueberries best)
Couple of ice cubes
Half a banana, fresh or frozen (optional, none on Reboot)
Greens (optional)
Yogurt or kefir
Protein powder if you like
Colon formula (1 scoop)
Little bit of water

Green Drink (great afternoon pick me up)

Half an apple (cut out core and chop coarsely, no need to peel)
Handful of chopped kale
Handful of chopped carrots (1 in. pieces)
Handful of chopped celery (1 in. pieces)
1/4 cucumber chopped (1 in. pieces)
Handful of chopped parsley
Piece of ginger root to taste, turmeric if desired
Any left over salad or other greens
Optional: a small beet, lightly cooked is best for some (raw kinda foams up and is stronger)
Optional: you can try adding small amounts of cabbage, broccoli or whatever else in refrig.
Coconut water or splash juice or kombucha
Water to just below fill line

Red Drink (Carrot/Beet/Ginger Drink)

Two handfuls carrots
1-2 beets, cooked
Ginger root, 1/2 inch slice peeled
Handful of mixed berries
Half an apple
Splash of cranberry or kombucha
Coconut water and or water

You can also add a small handful of kale if you like to make it more nutritious

V8 Type Drink

Two organic fresh tomatoes
Handful of celery
Handful of carrots
Whatever else you like, kale, lettuce, beans, cabbage (little bit of whatever)
Few ice cubes
Water or coconut water to just below fill line
Splash of hot sauce (optional)

APPENDIX C:
RECIPE SAMPLER & IDEAS TO INSPIRE YOU

The internet is full of great, easy and healthy recipes at your fingertips by entering in a few ingredients you want to use. Or you can buy a few healthy cookbooks.

Some of my favorite recipes are included here to get you started and spark your imagination. Healthy eating does not have to be boring!

Spinach & Feta Frittata

1 small bunch of spinach (or small package)

1/2 large onion

3 oz. feta or goat cheese

6 eggs

3 TBS parmesan/cheddar mix

1 TBS olive oil

2 garlic cloves minced

pinch of salt and fresh ground pepper

Preheat oven to 350 degrees. Heat oven proof skillet and add oil. Add minced garlic and onion and stir fry until translucent on medium heat. Add the fresh spinach and toss until wilted. Add the eggs, feta, salt and pepper and mix well. Top with grated parmesan and cheddar cheese and bake in oven until set. (serves 6)

Mexican Egg Scramble

6 eggs beaten

pinch of salt and fresh ground pepper

2 TBS water

1/2 TBS butter

3 green onions chopped

1 tomato chopped

3 TBS of diced cheddar cheese

Beat the eggs with the water. Heat a skillet and add butter, then eggs and lower heat gently tossing eggs over on top of each other from side until almost cooked. Add the green onions and cheddar cheese and stir into eggs. When cheese is almost melted, add the chopped tomato, toss and serve. (serves 3)

Crustless Broccoli and Cheddar Quiche

1 cup of finely chopped broccoli

1/2 white onion

3/4 cup cheddar cheese shredded

6 eggs

1/2 cup half and half

1 TBS butter

salt and pepper

Preheat oven to 350 degrees. Melt butter in skillet over medium heat. Add the chopped onion and cook until translucent. Add broccoli and quickly toss. Place the broccoli and onion in bottom of a well buttered quiche pan. Add pinch of salt and pepper to eggs and beat lightly adding the half and half. Pour over the broccoli and onion and top with the cheddar cheese. Bake until set and lightly browned on top, around 50 minutes. (serves 6)

Breakfast Tofu Bowl with Avocados

1 package extra firm tofu, drained well on towels

1 avocado, sliced

2 TBS olive oil

2 finely minced garlic cloves

1/2 finely chopped small red onion (in 2 portions)

2 Roma tomatoes, chopped finely

1 tsp onion powder

1 tsp garlic powder

1/4 tsp tumeric

1/4 tsp cumin

Salt and pepper to taste

1/2 can drained black beans

Juice of 1 lime or lemon

2 TBS chopped fresh cilantro

Hot sauce

Chop tofu into 1/2 in pieces. Heat fry pan with oil and add garlic and 1/2 the onion. Stir together 1 minute. Add tofu with onion powder, garlic powder and tumeric. Cook several minutes until tofu starts to brown and get crispy. In saucepan, sauce remainder of onion in 1 TBS olive or avocado oil until translucent. Add tomatoes and cook until reduced in liquid, about 3 minutes. Add black beans and salt and pepper. Stir for 1 minute, then add this to the tofu in fry pan and toss. Drizzle with lime or lemon. Serve in bowl over sliced avocados and top with fresh cilantro. Serve hot sauce on side. (serves 2)

Warm Quinoa Salad

2 cup dry quinoa

2 TBS sliced green onion or chopped red onion

1/2 cup chopped fresh cucumber

6 artichoke hearts

3/4 cup chopped olives or Mediterranean mix

Chopped sun dried tomatoes

Vegetable or chicken broth (optional)

4 TBS virgin olive oil

4 TBS balsamic vinegar

Cook the quinoa as directed optionally using broth instead of water. Set aside. Chop all other ingredients together and mix well. Mix olive oil and balsamic vinegar well adding any other herbs you like. Mix the olive mixture into quinoa and stir in the dressing.

Place clean salad greens on a plate and top with the quinoa mix. Leftover quinoa can be eaten cold with or without greens. (serves 6)

Chopped Mixed Veggie Salad

1 zucchini, diced into 1/2 in pieces

1 carrot, finely diced

1 onion, chopped finely

1 cucumber, diced into 1/2 in pieces

3 Roma tomatoes, chopped

1 can of marinated artichoke hearts, chopped

1/2 can heart of palm chopped (optional)

1 firm ripe avocado diced

2 TBS high quality virgin olive oil

Juice of one lime

2 TBS balsamic vinegar

Fresh 1 tsp finely chopped herbs (like rosemary, basil parsley or mint, optional)

Combine all veggie ingredients and mix well. Sprinkle with fresh lime juice and toss. Add olive oil, salt and pepper, fresh herbs and balsamic vinegar and toss again. (serves 4)

Roasted Veggie Bake

1 medium zucchini

1 onion

2 carrots

1 cup green beans in 2 in. pieces

1 cup sliced green cabbage

1 cup eggplant cut in 1 in. slices then large cubes

Any other veggies you wish to add

6 TBS minced garlic

Olive oil as needed for coating

2 cups chopped fresh tomatoes

1 can garbanzo beans

Salt and pepper to taste

Using a large skillet or wok, pour 2 TBS olive oil into pan and add 2 TBS of garlic, add vegetables divided in 3 batches for quickly stir frying with garlic and oil. Place vegetables into a large casserole dish in layers. Add the garbanzo beans and dash of salt and pepper and mix. Finally mix in the chopped tomatoes and bake in 350 degree oven for 50 minutes or until it is starting to just brown on top. Enjoy! (serves 6)

Mediterranean Green Beans with Garlic and Fresh Tomatoes

(serve warm or cold - a great potluck dish)

2 lbs. green beans chopped into 1.5 in. pieces

3 TBS minced garlic

2 cups chopped fresh ripe tomatoes

4 TBS olive oil

Use large skillet or wok, heat oil, then add garlic and green beans, stir frying on medium heat for 3 minutes. Add the chopped tomatoes, cover and simmer until the tomatoes are cooked down and beans are coated and cooked but still firm. Serve warm or cold. (serves 6)

Red Lentil Soup

(cooks in 1/2 hr., good with dollop of plain yogurt)

2 cups dried red lentils
1/2 chopped onion
1 TBS olive oil
1/2 TBS chopped garlic
1 Box of organic vegetable or chicken broth
Juice of 1/4 lemon
1/4 cup finely chopped tomato or TBS unsweetened ketchup

Rinse lentils in strainer. Heat oil in large saucepan and add garlic and onion. Cook over medium high heat for 2-3 minutes. Add the lentils and broth, cover and bring to boil. Simmer for 30 minutes, stirring occasionally and adding a bit of water if needed for a soup consistency. Add the chopped tomatoes (or ketchup) for last 15 minutes to add bit of color and sweetness. Serve with lemon squeeze and dollop of unsweetened yogurt. (serves 4)

Grilled Veggie & Chicken Skewers (Veggies can be a side dish served with veggie protein like barbecued seitan or tofu)

3 large chicken breasts sliced in 3/4 in. slices

Vegetables for roasting of your choice (green or yellow peppers, zucchini slices, carrots, cherry tomatoes, onion wedges)

Marinade of 2 fresh lemons juiced, 1/2 cup of unsweetened plain yogurt, and 1/4 cup of olive oil

1 Sprig of fresh rosemary, finely chopped

Mix marinade ingredients, add touch of salt and divide into two bowls. Add the chicken to one, the veggies to the other and toss to coat. Let sit for 2 hours in refrig. Soak bamboo skewers in water for 30 minutes or use metal skewers. Put chicken on some and veggies on other and either barbecue or grill under broiler until done and starting to brown slightly. (Serves 6 with a side dish like cauliflower coleslaw.)

Quick Broccoli Soup

1 small head of broccoli chopped small
1/2 large white onion
1 TBS olive oil
4 cups of broth (chicken or veggie)
salt and pepper

Heat a saucepan with oil. Add onion and sauté until translucent. Add broccoli and salt and pepper and toss in oil quickly. Add broth and simmer until broccoli is cooked, about 5 minutes. Blend in a blender or food processor until smooth. (serves 3-4)

Shredded Oriental Cabbage Salad

1 small shredded cabbage
1 bunch cilantro chopped
Chopped fresh snow peas
1 bunch green onions
1 bag slivered almonds
4 TBS toasted sesame seeds
salt and pepper to taste

Dressing

Equal parts sesame oil (or hot chili sesame oil) and tamari, start with 2 TBS each, add more if you wish

Mix, toss and serve. You may top with half a package of dried crunchy noodles like top ramen if you want some more interest to dish although it will not be as healthy. (serves 4-6)

Fast & Easy Black Bean Salad

2 cans black beans, rinsed and drained

1/2 cup chopped green onion

4 roma tomatos chopped

1 bunch cilantro, finely chopped

1 cup frozen corn

1 can chopped water chestnuts, rinsed and drained

1 firm avocado cubed in 3/4 in. pieces

Dressing

2 TBS olive oil, 2 TBS balsamic vinegar, dash of salt and pepper, and juice of one lime.

Mix, toss with dressing and serve over plate of greens with veggie chips and dollop of whole milk plain yogurt. (serves 4)

Mustard Butter Pasta with Broccoli

5/8 c butter or olive oil

4 TBS Dijon mustard

2 garlic cloves

2 TBS parsley, minced

2 TBS chives or green onion sliced

salt and pepper

2 c broccoli, cut small

¾ lb rice, amaranth or quinoa pasta (or zucchini spirals)

Blend oil with mustard. Pound garlic with pinch salt. Add parsley & chives. Blend with butter with black pepper.

Boil water, add pasta, partially cook and add broccoli for last two minutes of cooking. (Don't overcook rice pasta!) Toss all together and enjoy! (serves 3-4)

Asian Style Fish Stew

1 sweet potato

4 leaves red kale

2 Tbsp. olive oil

2 clove garlic, minced

1 large zucchini

2 cups veggie broth, low sodium

1/2 tsp. salt (or to taste)

1 tsp. lime zest

1/4 tsp. chili flakes

1 large leek

1 pound mahimahi or other white fish fillet, cut into bite-size
pieces

1 can coconut milk

1 Tbsp. lime juice, 1/2 bunch fresh cilantro, finely chopped

Peel the sweet potato and dice. Cut leek into diagonal slices
and rinse and chop the kale leaves into 1/2 in. slivers. Heat olive
oil in a saucepan and quickly sauté garlic. Add the chopped sweet
potato, sea salt, lime zest and chili flakes, and continue to sauté
for a couple of minutes.

Add broth to the veggies and bring to a boil. Cover and
simmer for about 5 minutes, then add the zucchini and leek and
continue to simmer for 5 minutes. Add the fish and coconut milk,
and simmer until the fish is almost cooked through, about 3 to
5 minutes. Add the chopped kale and continue to simmer for 4
minutes. Drizzle with lime juice and top with chopped cilantro.

Creamy Green Veggie Soup

1 cup onion, chopped

5 cloves garlic, chopped

2 tablespoons olive oil

2 cups zucchini, roughly chopped

2 cups yellow squash, roughly chopped

¼ cup celery, chopped

4 cups broccoli, chopped

4 cups green beans, cut into 1/2 in. pieces

8 cups veggie or chicken broth

2 large sprigs of fresh rosemary, finely chopped

½ teaspoon salt, fresh pepper to taste

Heat oil in large saucepan and cook onion and garlic until translucent over medium heat. Add celery, zucchini and squash and cook for 4 minutes. Add remaining vegetables, both and rosemary and simmer over low for 20 minutes. Puree in batches in your blender or with immersion blender. Serve with chopped rainbow salad. (serves 4-6)

Quick Cauliflower Coconut Stew

2 tablespoons coconut oil

1 teaspoon cumin seeds

1 medium onion, finely chopped

3 ripe tomatoes, finely chopped

1 medium head cauliflower, stemmed and cut into bite-size florets

1 jalapeno, stemmed, seeded, chopped

1 cup chopped kale

1 teaspoon finely chopped fresh ginger

2 tsp tablespoon cumin powder

2 tsp coriander powder

1/2 teaspoon turmeric powder

1 can full-fat, unsweetened coconut milk

1/2 teaspoon sea salt

2 TBS chopped cilantro

Heat coconut oil in medium saucepan. Add cumin seeds and stir for a minute, then add onions and cook until translucent. Add tomato and cook for another minute. Add rest of ingredients except cilantro, stir together and simmer over low heat about 15-20 minutes, stirring occasionally to prevent sticking. Serve with chopped cilantro. (serves 4)

Easy Butternut Squash Soup

1 butternut squash, peeled and cubed
1 large white onion, sliced
4 TBS butter
6 cups veggie stock
salt and pepper to taste
1 TBS fresh parsley, finely chopped

Heat large saucepan and add butter to melt. Add onion and cook over medium low heat until translucent and bit browned. Add the squash and toss, then add stock, cover and simmer until soft. Puree in blender or with immersion blender. Garnish with parsley.

Cauliflower Mashed Potatoes with Garlic

1 head cauliflower

2 TBS butter

2 TBS milk or unsweetened nut milk

Salt and pepper to taste

Very finely minced or fresh grated garlic to taste (2 cloves)

Chop cauliflower into florets and cook until tender in small amount of water with 1/2 tsp salt. Drain well and mash in pan with potato masher until creamy adding the butter, milk garlic and salt and pepper. (serves 4)

Sweet Potatoes with Spinach & Garlic

3 med sweet potatoes or yams, diced into 1 inch pieces

1 small bunch or 1 package spinach, chopped coarsely

3 TBS coconut oil

3 large cloves garlic, finely chopped

Salt and pepper to taste

Bring 4 cups water and 1 tsp salt to boil and parboil the potatoes until cooked but still firm. Drain and set aside. When ready to serve, heat the oil in fry pan, add the garlic and cook 2 minutes over medium heat. Add spinach and quickly stir fry the spinach until it begins to wilt. Add potatoes, stir about 2 minutes until heated, add salt and pepper to taste and serve. (serves 5-6)

Cauliflower Coleslaw

3/4 head of cauliflower, very finely chopped

1/4 head small cabbage (red or green) shredded

1 medium carrot, coarsely shredded

2 TBS healthy mayo

2 TBS vinegar (I prefer balsamic but rice vinegar is OK)

1 TBS virgin olive oil

Salt and pepper to taste

Whip together dressing ingredients in large bowl. Add veggies slowly mixing as you add them. Salt and pepper to taste. Best if it sits in refrig for hour or so. (serves 6)

Cauliflower Pizza (Not during Reboot)

1 head cauliflower, cut into florets or package cauliflower riced

3/4 cup mozzarella cheese

1 egg

2 TBS parmesan cheese

1/4 tsp salt and pepper

Red pizza sauce of your choice

Veggie toppings, your choice

Additional cheese to sprinkle on top

Cook cauliflower until tender and chop in food processor until just riced. (Don't over process!). Let cool a bit, squeeze out any water, then add parmesan cheese, mozzarella cheese and egg. Mix and spread out on baking pan or pizza pan lined with parchment paper and well oiled. Bake 15 min or until starting to brown at 425 degrees.

Meanwhile chop and prepare toppings. Spread sauce evenly over pizza, place toppings on it and small amount of additional cheese if you like. Bake at 425 degrees or until starting to brown a bit. Let sit 10 min. Enjoy!

Fresh Pineapple with Champagne

1 ripe pineapple, diced into 1 in pieces

Champagne to cover

2 TBS unsweetened grated coconut

Chop pineapple and drizzle the champagne over it. Let it sit in refrig covered for several hours. Serve with a topping of the coconut. Enjoy. (serves 6)

Creamy Dairy Free Chocolate Mousse

2 bananas

1 ripe avocado

1/4 c unsweetened cocoa powder

1 TBS honey or stevia to taste (30 drops)

Blend the bananas and avocado in food processor until creamy and smooth. Add cocoa powder and process. Add honey and or stevia to taste. Chill well in individual serving bowls. Top with a dollop of whip cream or yogurt alternative to make it extra special. *(This can be made with no sweeteners at all and is still very tasty!)*

Bullet Style Coffee

3/4 cup good coffee (like mine pretty strong)
1 TB Butter
1 TBS Coconut Oil

Make coffee, add butter and coconut and blend oil frothy. Enjoy

Homemade Ginger Ale

1/2 cup finely chopped ginger, peeled
3 cups water
Juice of 4 fresh limes
2 TBS Coconut nectar sweetener, honey, or 20 drops stevia (Sweet Leaf)

Peel and chop ginger. A small spice chopper works great. Add to 3 cups water in saucepan and simmer 15 minutes on low. Strain well, add lime juice, and sweetener of your choice. Pour into a glass storage bottle and refrigerate. To serve pour about an inch of syrup over ice in tall glass, add splash of other fresh fruit juice if desired and fill with soda water.

APPENDIX D: RESOURCE GUIDE

MORE INFO ON FOOD, SUPPLEMENTS AND RECIPES

ONLINE INFORMATION RESOURCES:

www.functionalmedicine.org

www.dietdoctor.com/low-carb

www.drhyman.com (loads of info on most everything)

www.nutritionaltypedrmercola.com

www.doctoroz.com/article/10-day-detox-diet-one-sheet

www.vegetarian.org

www.draxe.com (intestinal health info, healing leaky gut and other GI issues)

INFORMATIONAL BOOKS:

Grain Brain by Dr. David Perlmutter, MD

The Coconut Diet by Cherie Calbom and John Calbot

Eat Fat, Get Thin by Dr. Mark Hyman

The Blood Sugar Solution by Dr. Mark Hyman

The South Beach Diet by Arthur Agastston, MD

Wired to Eat by Rob Wolf

The Paleo Diet by Loren Cordain, PhD

Paleo Diet: Paleo for Beginners - How to Eat Like a Caveman and Get Leaner, Stronger and More Energetic! by Sarah E. Dawson

Diet for a New America by John Robbins

How to Be a Vegetarian by Rex Henderson

The Third Plate by Dan Barber

The Forks Over Knives Plan by Alona Pulde M.D. and Matthew Lederman M.D.

RECIPE BOOKS:

The Low Carb High Fat Cookbook: 100 Recipes to Lose Weight and Feel Great by Dana Campbell

The Eat Fat, Get Thin Cookbook by Dr. Mark Hyman

Eat Complete by Drew Ramsey, MD

The Ketogenic Cookbook: Nutritous Low-Carb, High Fat Paleo Meals to Heal Your Body by Jimmy Moore

Low Carb, High Fat Food Revolution to Improve Your Health and Reduce Your Weight by Andreas Eenfedt

The Everything Coconut Diet Cookbook by Anji Sandage & Lorena Novak Bull, RN

Low Carb High Fat Cooking for Healthy Aging: 70 Easy and Delicious Recipes to Promote Vitality and Longevity by Annika Dahlqvist Birgitta Hglund

The Mindfulness Cookbook by Dr. Patricia Collard & Helen Stephenson

The Uncook Book by Tanya Mayer

The Part-time Vegetarian, Flexible Recipes To Go (Nearly meat-free) by Nicola Graines

The Thousand Recipe Chinese Cookbook by Gloria Bly Miller

Crazy Sexy Kitchen by Kris Carr and Chef Chad Sarno

Vegetarian Times Cookbook by editor Lucy Moll

Make Your Own Rules Cookbook by Tara Stiles

Naturally Sassy by Saskia Gregson-Williams

Paleo Monday to Friday by Daniel Green

I Quit Sugar - Simplicious by Sarah Wilson (306 sugar-free recipes)

The South Beach Diet Quick & Easy Cookbook by Arthur Agatston, MD

"May all beings, all persons be blessed with good health, happiness, prosperity and spirituality."

— **Grand Master Choa Kok Sui**

A special thanks to my editor Suzanne MacLeod and all of the health practitioners out there working to change our beliefs about food and help us all find a way of eating healthy that works and improves out quality of health. Together we can make a difference, one life, one family at a time!

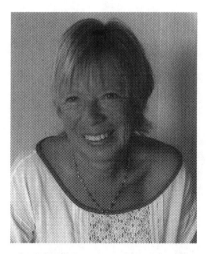

Cyndy graduated with a Masters in Pharmacy from the University of Washington in 1972. After working in a community pharmacy for several years, she came to believe that if she was going to achieve her goal of making a real difference in people's lives, conventional medicine and pharmaceuticals might not offer the best solutions. Her first "Integrative" certification was in hypnotherapy, building a large private practice in Hood River, Oregon. Cyndy developed a special passion for dietary wellness counseling and various forms of energy healing work, in addition to the use of hypnotherapy, eventually developing a unique program based on 'feeding a hungry heart'.

The inspiration for this book came after a serious auto accident which left her unable to do the things she loved. Hiking, swimming and gardening were lost to her because of neck and back injuries. A debilitating TBI (concussive injury) caused memory loss and loss of basic cognitive processing, verbal communication and social skills. The effects on her life were profound and compounded by PTSD and frequent severe anxiety attacks. She set out on a path of self healing. Along the way, she decided to put her life-long acquired knowledge about healthy eating and its importance into a book.

Recently she served as the wellness consultant at a cutting edge regenerative medicine clinic in Roatan, Honduras. She now lives in Palm Springs offering lectures, classes and individual session work on dietary wellness and hypnotherapy. She also teaches tai chi. Her web site is healyourlife.info.

Printed in the United States
by Baker & Taylor Publisher Services